Revolt of
The Stomach

Phlegm Mass Disorder:
The Cause of All Diseases

Seo Hyung Choi

Revolt of the Stomach

Phlegm Mass Disorder: The Cause of All Diseases

Authored by Seo Hyung Choi
Translated by Choon Taeck Kong

Copyright © 2017 by Seo Hyung Choi
ISBN-13: 978-1545310892
ISBN-10: 1545310890

All rights reserved. Under International Copyright Law, no part of this book may be reproduced or transmitted in any form or by any means, electronic or mechanical-including photocopying, recording, or by any information storage and retrieval system- without permission in writing from the author. Please direct your inquiries to hana9212@korea.com.

Table of Contents

Preface 7

How Has This Book Come Into Being? 9

Part 01 Unknown Cause Gastrointestinal Tract Disorder Endoscopy Cannot Detect

1. Pain is killing me, but you call it 'neurogenic?' 16
2. Look for the cause hidden in the word 'neurogenic'! 18
3. Koreans with wellbeing foods — Stomach cancer incidence #1 in the world? 22

Part 02 The Stomach Knows!

1. What 700 people have in common whose endoscopy reading shows normal but still feeling pain? 26
2. Koreans' way of handling the stomach 31

Part 03 Middle Zone – the Gastrointestinal Tract Part Endoscopy Cannot See

1. New discovery of the stomach of 0.1 to 0.3 inch width! 36

2. Cutting edge Head Quarters that are hidden behind the mucous membrane 38

3. Middle Zone – hidden treasure in the gastrointestinal tract 45

4. Why isn't the sick stomach detected in the endoscopy? 47

Part 04 True Nature of Gastrointestinal Tract Disorder Revealed

1. Indigestion, obvious symptoms, but no reason? 54

2. Mucous membrane gate, the guard of our body 55

3. Cause of mucous membrane damage, everything! 57

4. Middle Zone damage that leads to hardening of outer wall of gastrointestinal tract 69

5. Gastrointestinal tract disorder that has symptoms but no causes: 'Phlegm Mass Disorder' 74

6. The reality of phlegm mass disorder 75

Part 05 Phlegm Mass Disorder Leads to Cirrhosis, Diabetes

1. Disorder in Middle Zone, the septic tank of our body, leads to the pollution of the whole body 90

2. Change of whole body caused by phlegm mass disorder 92

3. Major retractable diseases caused by phlegm mass disorder 96

Part 06 Diagnosis and Treatment of Phlegm Mass Disorder

1. Treatment of phlegm mass disorder 124
2. Our body can be improved this much when phlegm mass disorder treated 132

Part 07 Silencing the Revolt of the Stomach

1. Time to examine our unusual eating habits! 142
2. Foods and eating habits that easily cause phlegm mass disorder 144
3. Health care guide that silences all diseases 146

Appendix

I treated my gastrointestinal tract disorder this way 155

Preface

Endoscopy reading shows no defect. Having symptom but no known cause of stomach trouble?

Having stomach trouble, seeing doctor, however, one has no known trouble even after endoscopy. Therefore, one is diagnosed as having 'neurogenic stomach disease.' It is the disease that has obvious symptoms but has no solution and is called chronic neurogenic gastrointestinal tract disorder! Now, let us look at outer wall of the gastrointestinal tract. Over there, more serious diseases are developing, worse than mucous disease, such as gastritis, and gastric ulcer. With the finding of 'phlegm mass disorder', the deteriorating of outer wall of stomach, we see the solution to the curiosity and suffering of the disorder.

People of nowadays are living with stomach with broken emergency alarm.

Overeating causes indigestion and feeling bloated and discomfort. Do you know that it is better to feel that way?

Stomach has an alarm system that can protect itself by expressing various digestive symptoms. But nowadays, people's stomach emergency bell for the most part went wrong and is not working properly. People boast about their stomach that they would feel OK no matter how much and how fast they eat. Their stomach is strong and they become confident of their health. But do not boast! It is simply because your emergency bell got broken. Big diseases are developing in your body.

What is all the fuss about stomach disease? The used to be 'quiet stomach' begins the revolt!

People of long enduring personality may explode to anger once prompted. Stomach does explode after being treated as 'food container' (stomach and 'food container' are homonym in Korean) for a long time. Because of all the engulfed food, the 'food container' succumbs to phlegm mass disorder and its poisons spread to the whole body, such as, liver, heart, brain, skin, and joints. The stomach disease has become breeding ground of all diseases. We cannot treat stomach as 'food container' anymore.

How Has This Book Come Into Being?

It was after experiencing lots of failures and frustrations that I became aware of exterior wall of stomach causing stomach disorder, not the mucous membrane of stomach. My clinical research was on liver and stomach and I saw many a chronic stomach disorder patients. Those skinny patients, being unable to eat, could not even swallow medicine no matter how excellent it meant to be and therefore often ended in failure. Underneath their shallow abdomen skin, I could usually detect stony hard organs, moving separate from the skin. It was clearly not the abdomen fat or muscle layer but felt painful when pressed. Endoscopy does not show defects inside. Abdomen CT does not detect it a cancer. In the beginning, I did not think that it was hardened part of exterior wall of stomach. Because of those patients, I began conducting epidemiologic survey over the severe indigestion cases. Wonju Biomedical Research Institute invented a device that measures the hardened part of exterior wall of stomach. Applying the technic, I became confident that the hardened part was truly exterior part of stomach. I have named this new concept of disorder 'phlegm mass disorder' and developed new medicines accordingly. As a result, after taking those medicines, patients felt their stomach move and were able to eat. Existing treatments did not work to them previously.

Being a clinician, I leapt for joy. It means that neurogenic and functional gastrointestinal tract disorder, the hard to diagnose disorders, has something to do with external wall of stomach and intestines. For what else could I be more joyous than this?

Then the joy stopped soon when I encountered the question, 'why does it get hardened?' There are hardened organs, I said, but I could not answer to 'why?' From there I started examining the inner organs hidden underneath the mucous membrane by looking up the most recent studies. It was about why and how that part becomes badly changed. Once opened, that part of our body displayed incredible amount of organisms and functions that are beyond our imagination. Moreover, the stomach and intestines filled me with awe when I noticed the wisdom and patience they show in protecting our body from influx of harmful substances. It was no less than a mystery. I named this book 'the revolt of the stomach' as an irony in an effort of awakening our ignorance; we have mistreated stomach and intestines so much.

I named the external mucous wall of stomach and intestines 'Middle Zone' to imply that it is in the center of our body. I also named the damaged and swollen middle zone 'phlegm mass disorder.' With the discovery of middle zone and phlegm mass disorder, the spectrum of gastrointestinal tract diseases widened. Its treatments will also be renewed. Since the middle zone is where the absorbed nutrition is decomposed and distributed throughout the body, once damaged, it becomes the breeding ground of innumerous diseases of our body. The implication of this knowledge has become significant. Accumulated phlegm mass toxin in the middle zone spread over the whole body through blood vessels and lymph and causes diabetes, cirrhosis, hardening of the arteries, various autoimmune disorders, skin diseases such as atopy, rheumatic arthritis, dizziness, and dementia. This has been confirmed through the process of diagnosis and treatment of the patients. We therefore have to watch carefully how phlegm mass disorder and whole body diseases are closely related. Further studies need to be done on how engulfing food, gluttony, overeating, and food toxin affect the middle zone, and how it influences starting of diseases. As petroleum based industry and pollution of water and soil have made our dining no longer safe, the study on how food and disease are related become critically important medical mandate.

Since phlegm mass disorder is the breeding ground of diseases of whole body, its treatment is more fundamental because it deals with the root of problems. Modern medicine, however, tends to focus on symptoms and improving phenomena. Removing of symptom is easy and so is the recurring of the disease, because the body is not yet changed. It is far more important to improve the environment of the disease than treatment of symptoms or phenomena. This is true medicine that deals with fundamentals of our body to remove diseases.

While treating phlegm mass disorder, I had a patient recognize what true medicine was. It is the story of a 28 year-old female patient who came to complain about her severe acne, dizziness, general fatigue, and depression. Diagnosing the severe phlegm mass disorder, I treated the toxin for about 2 weeks and heard her saying that her acne had relieved, headache and dizziness disappeared and whole body became improved, but indigestion started. She said that she had been very confident of digesting food. When stressed, she used to engulf much food, ate noodles before going to bed, but had no problem in digestion, she claimed. But after she got treated in this clinic, she could feel a little bit more food cause immediate indigestion problem. Upon hearing that, I said, 'your stomach started function healthy. Your whole body will become healthy. So do not worry about it.' I added that 'once you feel indigestion, it is the sign that you should stop eating. Control your food then'

That is it! The patient's indigestion is the healthy response to the overeating, to protect her body. The treatment fixed the deformed response of stomach and intestine to be of healthy one. Likewise, true medicine should improve the body so as to respond healthy and correctly and teach people to comply with such lifestyle.

This book underscores the integral role of the gastrointestinal tract and its maintenance to lifelong physical wellbeing. It also serves to remind us that neglecting health by not paying attention to the food which enters our systems may cause irreparable damage to the stomach as well as to the body. It not only advises on gastrointestinal tract system management but also on how to reverse the damage from disease and systemic harm due to bad habits. The core messages of this book can be boiled down to the following 4 points.

Firstly, the neurogenic, functional gastrointestinal tract disorder, that has been difficult to diagnose and therefore hard to treat, is actually because of the damaged 'middle zone' of mucous outer wall of the stomach.

Secondly, various causes may destroy the protective measures of mucosal outer wall of stomach and intestine. I called this finding 'the most important event' in the medical history. It is because, once the protective shield of gastrointestinal tube is destroyed, the innumerous poisonous substances that have entered the stomach and intestine can spread throughout the whole body and cause many kinds of diseases.

Thirdly, lots of hard to treat chronic diseases, because of its causes and pathological mechanisms are not clear, have something to do with phlegm mass disorder.

Fourthly, the most typical cause of damage of mucosal gastrointestinal protective shield is the bad habit of eating and intake of poisonous food. Therefore, improving one's diet is crucial.

While this resource is not a medical journal, it is written to spread the fact that lots of diseases come into being from bad eating habits. It is also intended to make known the reality of chronic and neurogenic gastrointestinal tract diseases. This writer intends to further research on the implications of phlegm mass disorder and thus contributes toward the prevention and treatment of many diseases through improving daily diets.

In addition, there were difficult issues for general readers to understand, because of the jargons of pathologies and the nature of gastrointestinal tract diseases. It took lots of time to make it easily readable. For that, many thanks go to the two writers; Hyun Ju Jung and Ji Young Eun.

Seo Hyung Choi

Part 01

Unknown Cause Gastrointestinal Tract Disorder Endoscopy Cannot Detect

1

Pain is killing me, but you call it 'neurogenic?'

'I always feel bloated and full of gas inside.'
'I feel my pit of the stomach blocked and suffocating.'
'Once stressed, my stomach almost always gets upset.'
'Feeling poked by needle and so awfully painful.'

People with stomach diseases commonly share these words. Being Suspicious of contracting big disease, they may undergo various tests, e.g., stomach endoscopy, colon endoscopy, but only hear that nothing is serious. They will likely hear another ambiguous word, i.e., 'It is just neurogenic nature. Therefore, relax and forget about it, you will then get better.' The pain almost kills. How can you possibly forget it? For a patient, it is so embarrassing to hear such words all the time. On one hand, the patient feels fortunate not to have dreadful diseases such as cancer or ulcer. But on the other hand, not many diseases are more ambiguous and hard to cure than neurogenic stomach disease. Though feeling heartburn and painful, one has no tangible endoscopy result in the stomach. It suggests that there is no need to treat, or cannot even treat. Among 476 walk in patients, only 19% (90 people) had organic cause according to 'Rome standard III', the functional digestive disorder index, and the 81% (386 people) had no organic cause of the disease, according to the medical institutes of Korea. Simply put, when people undergo endoscopy on account of indigestion, 7 or 8 out of 10 people will find no clue of the problem.

What are the reasons of Koreans' stomach becoming more troublesome, showing no special problems on stomach endoscopy but having various symptoms such as, pain on the pit of the stomach, convulsion, bloating, heartburn, burping, vomiting, reflux, and stomach upset?

TIP: Any Koreans would experience, 'heartburn'

Feeling sharp, aching, scratching, poking, tearing, sting

When skin peeled off and medicine applied to it, we feel burning and pain. Heartburn is like the skin burn feeling. It takes place when mucous membrane or epithelial cell get cracked and stomach acid or any irritating substance reaches the nerve under epithelium. Heartburn causing diseases are reflux esophagitis, medicine caused esophagitis, erosive gastritis, gastric ulcer, duodenal ulcer, stomach cancer, pregnancy caused reflux. It happens, for the most part, that increased stomach acid irritates weakened epithelial tissue and make it aching.

2

Look for the causes hidden in the 'neurogenic' nature!

When one feels pain but can't find the causes, the name 'neurogenic' is given. As is the most neurogenic diseases, there is no fundamental treatment of the trouble, and one tends to accept it as destiny. But they suffer more from the ambiguous nature of the problem, more than those who have known stomach diseases, such as ulcer.

One loses appetite, because of the indigestion, and the poor nutrition naturally leads to lowered energy, and it affects one's work and work morale declines, the evil cycle continues. But one's family and friends may say, 'what is all the fuss about? It is just neurogenic indigestion trouble anyway.' Doctors take it lightly and simply suggest that one has to relax and not worry too much. Therefore one gets even more irritated. In this sense, the diagnosis, 'neurogenic' is too irresponsible to stressful modern day people.

Neurogenic indigestion disorder, however, is not a simple disease that we can ignore and move on. Though its medical symptom may look small, the pain signals the bigger danger inside the body. The following case teaches us not to ignore such 'neurogenic stomach disorder.'

A woman in her late 50s, 5 feet 3 inches height, and 83lbs weight, came to see me. She had lost more than 33lbs in the last 2 or 3 years. She could not even swallow a cup of water by then. Since she could not eat at all, she had to live on IV nutrition in a university hospital. She felt that she must have contracted a big cancer, and therefore she underwent all kinds of tests relating to stomach. Each time, she heard that she had no problem. She could not have any way of treating, because she had no known disease to cure. The medicine she received had no effect on her either. She spent the life of suffering and anxiety.

Before she got ill, she worked as a street vendor. Since she could not eat on time, she had to hurriedly swallow rice with water. As I examined her belly, her whole abdomen part became as hard as stone. With this much stiffened organ, stomach activities were by no means possible and could not let the food content go down the intestine. However, endoscopy could not observe this stiffened stomach system. It was diagnosed simply as 'stomach, no problem.'

One more memorable patient was a 44 years old, successful Korean American businessman. Enjoying his happy life, he visited Korea to attend his nephew's wedding after a long absence. He decided to have a medical check in a university hospital, but knew that he had contracted a terminal stomach cancer. The unexpected always happens! One year before that, he had endoscopy in the States. It was a mild case of neurogenic gastritis. How could that develop to the terminal stomach cancer, he wondered?

He was a lover of good food. He just felt a bit stuffy in the pit of the stomach when overeating. He also felt something hard and a little bit of pain but never had indigestion problem. As with most of other patients do, he could not accept the test result and went from one hospital to another to examine further. It was the same terminal stomach cancer, and he had to struggle against extreme anxiety. He eventually died of cancer after six months and had his funeral in Korea without having to return to the States. Something serious was developing to stomach cancer, but endoscopy could not detect it.

TIP: Beating breast and cries out, 'feeling stuffy!'

Feeling full, feel like something got caught in my throat, feeling heavy, uncomfortable, stomach upset

Feeling stuffy means that something is blocked and not flowing down. Being blocked means that a process of communication to the brain through nervous system is needed. Feeling stuffy also means that the nerve endings in the stomach are sending signals to the brain.

When eating fast or overeating, the physical/chemical pressure given to any parts of pharynx, larynx, throat, stomach, or duodenum stimulates nerve endings and it reaches to the brain, and we feel 'stuffy.' The uncomfortable feeling is a healthy response to protect our body from food wastes or toxins that is caused by overdrinking, overeating, and fast eating. Sometimes we still feel stuffy without having such physical stimulants. It is when the capacity of swallowing food and make it go down becomes weak or because of stress one receives. For the stomach to make the food go down the intestine, liver's role is essential. Liver is to make nerves to have seamless communication and to energize secreting digestive enzymes. But once function of the liver freezes, caused by stress, neurohormone secreting system, operated by mutual communication between brain and liver, also freezes and strained.

3

Koreans with wellbeing food, Stomach cancer incidence #1 in the world

1 out of 4 male cancer patients and 1 out of 7 female cancer patients have stomach cancer, and therefore it is called 'national cancer.' Colon cancer was known as the westerners' cancer in the past, but it is now 2nd most frequent cancer, out-numbering liver cancer and lung cancer. Statistics points that it is a serious problem as much as to be called 'national disease.' Many scientists in the world acknowledge Kimchi, soybean paste, cheonggukjang (fast-fermented bean paste) as excellent anti-cancer fermented food and useful to stomach and intestine. But how can it be explained that Koreans, eating those anti-cancer food, have #1 stomach cancer incidence rate in the world? More surprisingly, there are more stomach cancer incidences in Korea than less developed nations where nutritional status and sanitary conditions are poor. Some people may argue that it is salty and spicy hot food that causes the problem. But some people in Europe or tropical regions enjoy more salty and spicy hot food. That food is not the only reason of the stomach cancer. Why do Koreans stand out in the malignant digestive disease incidence?

The stomach disorder: symptoms with no solutions! Koreans

with wellbeing foods but has stomach cancer incidence #1! In order to examine the cause of the Koreans' stomach disorder, the previous two patients' cases are mentioned again.

The two cases show the typical big gap between the result of endoscopy and actual suffering from stomach disorder. It is because of the limitation of endoscopy which examines only the mucous membrane of inside of stomach, and becomes the dilemma of digestive medical science. This dilemma, however, can find solution if we do not limit the examination to the reading of endoscopy, and open to the possibility of finding solution in some unknown area where endoscopy cannot detect.

Looking at the 3 dimensional structure of gastrointestinal tract, we easily find that mucous membrane that endoscopy examines occupies only a small part of entire stomach and intestines. On the exterior walls of stomach, not on the mucous membrane, there exist far more complex and diverse organs. This exterior walls is the 70 to 80 percent of the gastrointestinal tract area that endoscopy could not examine. This is also the place where fatal cancer may have developed without being noticed.

With this inference, the following epidemiologic survey was conducted to see on what parts troubles appear, besides mucous membrane, and to see any specific problems may happen.

Part 02

Stomach Knows!

1

What 700 people have in common whose endoscopy reading shows normal, but still feeling pain?

In 2003, Division of Gastroenterology team of Weedahm Oriental Hospital chose 700 patients who had complained severe gastrointestinal tract disease but their endoscopy reading looked normal, and investigated a few points. The research team used acoustic test and pressation to examine the extent of hardness, swelling, and pain of stomach and intestines, and classified into 12 stages according to the extent of pain and hardness. They also conducted a questionnaire to understand the whole body symptoms, such as on diet habits, favorite foods, complaining gastrointestinal tract symptoms, headaches, and skin symptoms. To examine also any malfunction of the stomach and intestine, using EAV (Electroacupuncture According to Voll) tester that tests the level of organ functions, we have come to the following recognition.

Palpation of abdomen result

In most cases, patients had stony hard stomach and intestine outer wall. When pressed, they complained severe pressure pain. The result was the same when abdomen muscle or fat layer of the abdomen were lifted aside and only stomach and intestine parts were palpated.

This hospital and Wonju Medical Science Institute were cooperatively developing a machine that measures the level of hardness of the stomach outer wall. Using the machine and examining, the same fact was confirmed that the hardened mass was the outer wall of stomach and intestine.

Oriental medicine EAV test reading

To observe the muscular strength, lymph condition, nerve and blood vessel functions, EAV tester applied, and we have come to know that the index level significantly dropped in stomach, small intestine, large intestine, and in duodenum. It means that with the influence of food toxins or other pathogenic factor, gastro-intestinal tract does not function properly.

Questionnaire reading

In order to know patients' daily eating habits, questionnaires were conducted, and we came to know that most of them had the habit of eating fast, and overeating. They were inclined to eating wheats or sensitive to wheats.

Many of the patients did not have time to eat, and therefore practically engulfed foods to eat fast, such as shoving in a spoonful of meats, while grasping another spoonful of meat with the other hand, and skipping meals but eating a lot all of a sudden. Eating at night before going to bed, eating mostly wheat products, such as

Ramen, bread, noodles, or swallowing rice with water, shows all the bad eating habits.

Whole body symptoms

Patients with stomach disorders, in many cases, have complex whole body symptoms. Questionnaires were conducted to see what kinds of symptoms accompany those with hardened outer walls of stomach and intestine. It turns out that many kinds of diseases appear, such as, headache, dizziness, vomiting impulse, shoulder ache, bad breath, freckles, pimples, chest pains, exhaustion, and uterine disease.

The following facts become common among the patients who appear normal in the endoscopy reading but complain severe gastrointestinal tract disorder symptoms:

1. Most patients habitually eat fast, eat heavy, and overeat.
2. Their outer wall of stomach and of intestine become hardened, feeling pain once pressed.
3. Swollen and hardened tissues are filled with toxins, and it spreads all over whole body to cause various kinds of diseases.

It has become obvious that among neurogenic stomach disorder patients, outer walls of their stomach and intestine become swollen and hardened because of their wrong eating habits, and therefore toxin environments are formed inside the gastrointestinal tract.

TIP: Eating over and over again, but feeling the sense of hunger!

Hungry, having eaten but still hungry, feeling empty stomach, feeling a little hungry, feeling hypoglycemia, feeling blue, not happy, not meeting expectation

Abnormal sense of hunger is when one has eaten enough, not yet even eating time, but still feels hungry. Among diabetes patients, feeling hunger is common when blood sugar depletes or its supply is not enough. Therefore, the feeling of hunger is more of metabolism disorder than of stomach disorder. Feeling hungry because of roundworm inside is also about metabolism of nutrition.

The pathological hunger because of stomach disorder sometimes accompanies heartburn, but it appears mostly because of abnormal response of intestine nervous system. To explain it simpler, when food intake is more than what one can digest, intestine nervous system discern the situation and send signal to brain to cause symptoms happen such as bloating, pain, vomiting, or diarrhea so that no more food would not come in, therefore it controls and protects. However, because of various reasons (mostly because of food toxins), intestine nerve degenerated, and it cannot discern the situation correctly, and send out wrong signal to the brain. The brain, in turn, secretes hunger hormone. One, then, gets easily hungry and feels empty stomach and therefore become compelled to overeat, and feels comfortable going to bed after eating food at late night. In this case, bigger problems appear in the body, such as diabetes, cancer, various metabolic syndromes, skin troubles, or stroke risk factors rise. One of the most important functions of the gastrointestinal tract nervous system is that when too much or poisonous foods are taken in, nervous system detects and sends signals to brain so that it causes pain, vomiting, bloating, or diarrhea and therefore protects our body from food hazards. Once nervous systems become degenerated, it does not detect it and therefore food poisons gush in and body remain unprotected and damaged.

2

Koreans' way of handling 'food container'

Stomach and food container are homonym in Korean.

As expected, epidemiological survey shows that Koreans' typical way of eating habit makes cancer incidence rate #1 in the world. It may also be the cause of chronic stomach disorder of which its reason is not known. With this in mind, we overview Koreans' eating culture.

Eating good food in big quantity is regarded the prime importance of health issue to Koreans

The greeting, 'How are you?' is not as sincere greeting as 'Have you eaten?' to Koreans. Eating well has naturally become the top virtue after experiencing 'the farm hardship period' of the past. Therefore, the nation regards eating as the most important virtue. No matter how much swallowed, once digested, it is the best way to the health, people think. They have eating oriented health view and nobody seems to teach or willing to know about how to eat properly. Eating good and well is enough, how can 'how to eat' become the issue to treat disease, people think? Medicines, therefore, neglect providing research and scientific information about how to eat. Doctors do not put emphasis on the issue either. Instead, eating becomes even more important when in sickness. Eating various health diets is further emphasized.

Koreans' treating stomach simply as 'food container'
(stomach and food container are homonym in Korean)

'Excuse me, bring me the food quick!' 'Excuse me, can you make it quick?'

These are the shouts we hear at every lunch hour in Yoido financial streets. I am sure that it is not limited to Yoido only. This is the very shout we hear right after clocks hit 12 o'clock all over the nation. It is said that the spirit of 'hurry, hurry' explains the reason why the nation Korea has achieved the brilliant economic growth in recent decades. However, as a medical doctor, I would say that this is the very reason why Koreans' stomach and general health turned downward.

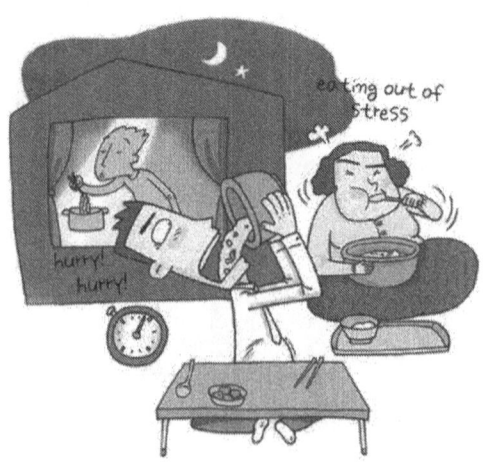

There are differences among individuals, but Koreans usually eat 3 times faster than people of other developed countries. People shove in foods without knowing what troubles it may entail and just believing that stomach would take care of everything.

No matter how late at night, without putting some food in stomach, one cannot make sleep. Therefore, one has to cook and eat noodles even at midnight. Stomach is also the object of venting one's anger on, mixing Bibimbob with crimson red spicy hot pepper paste on a big bowl, shoving in to the stomach. Not considering the nutrition values, people just throwing in any food, thinking that stomach would handle everything. Most of those people have no idea how those foods arrive in the stomach and what happen next. They think that what you eat is what you get, and that is what truly yours.

The dining habit of ours that treats gastrointestinal tract as just food container gradually ruins our digestion systems.

TIP: 'Gastric ulcer', the perpetual main character of TV commercials for husbands!

When mucous membrane becomes damaged in a deeper level, it is called 'erosive gastritis.' 'Erosive' means its surface is peeled off. When the root of the mucous membrane is damaged, it is called, 'gastric ulcer.' Erosive gastritis indicates that it is damaged up to mucous membrane, and gastric ulcer up to mucous membrane muscle. If blood vessels beneath the mucous membrane muscles are exposed, it may cause gastrorrhagia, the bleeding of stomach.

Stomach cancer develops by mucous cells mutation. Excessive increase of cancerous cells damage other organs. The mutation of mucous cells develops in connection to the organs of beneath the mucous membrane.

Are you becoming a bit nervous? 'Duodenal ulcer'

Duodenum is one of the major organs that digests and absorbs. In the process of digestion and absorption, mucous membrane damage can easily happen. It happens in the form of duodenitis or duodenal ulcer. Even without the infection on the organs, various symptoms of indigestions and discomforts may appear. It is easily understood if we think of how duodenum involves in various functions of digestion and absorption.

Jejunum of Small intestines deals with the absorption and feels no pain or hurt, and therefore it is not easy to detect accurate status. Infection of small intestines results mainly in diarrhea. It can't absorb, therefore it is to loose bowels.

Part 03
Middle Zone, the Gastrointestinal Tract Part Endoscopy Cannot See

1

New discovery of the stomach of 0.1 to 0.3 inch width

Gastrointestinal tract patients whose mucous membrane proved all right commonly show hardened organs with oppressive pain when palpating the outer wall of stomach. Wanting to find all the solution to the Koreans' stomach disorder, the one of 'obvious symptoms with no reason,' we begin to examine the outer wall tissue of mucous membrane.

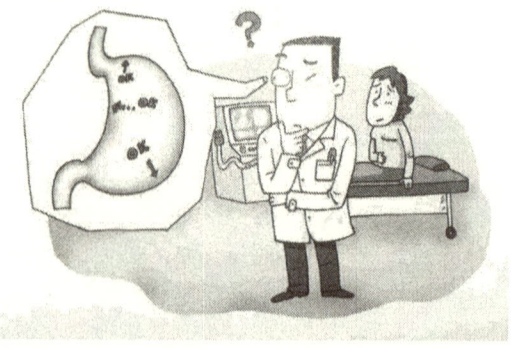

Imagine now that we receive endoscopy. Lying on the bed, one notices endoscope comes in through mouth. Once it passes the mouth and the airway, it slowly shows the inside on the monitor. Passing the throat which look like folded alleys, arriving in stomach, it shows the stomach in scarlet color. With the help of endoscope, doctors examine whether it has any wounds, hyperemia, bloodstain, or polyps. During the 5 to 10 minutes of examination, doctors' discernments are based on the visible sign of the mucous membrane. But the gastrointestinal tract endoscopy shows only the surface of mucous membrane of inside the stomach.

We now talk about the tissues, fivefold, consist of 0.1 to 0.3 inches width, outside of mucous membrane, not the mucous membrane surface of the gastrointestinal tract.

2
Cutting edge Head Quarters that are hidden behind the mucous membrane

It may vary from person to person, but stomach is made with five layers, 0.1 to 0.3 inches width 3 dimensional tissues. Intestines are thinner than this but have similar wall structure as the stomach. It has radiator like villus bumps to make absorption easy. Outside the mucous membrane, there exist extremely complex and detailed organs in the thin tissues.

In this zone, there is GALT (Gut Associated Lymphoid Tissue), the highly developed immune system of our body. There are endogenous nervous system that works inside the gastrointestinal tract, and exogenous nervous system that works in connection with brain and spinal cord. The immune system brags about vast amount of organisms. Nervous system here is installed far more, in number, than in spinal nervous system. In a word, the most elite military and intelligence system functions inside the gastrointestinal tract. The reason the Creator installed this much highly developed defense system is that gastrointestinal tract plays the most important role in defending our body healthy.

It is also equipped with hormone system that controls stomach activities and different enzyme secreting activities, and secretory organs that secrete digestion promoting enzymes and gastrointestinal tract protecting slime substance, and muscle systems that mix and push the foods down, and vessel networking system through which nutrition and energy are provided between gastrointestinal tract and whole body. It is hard to fathom all the functions with our human capacity.

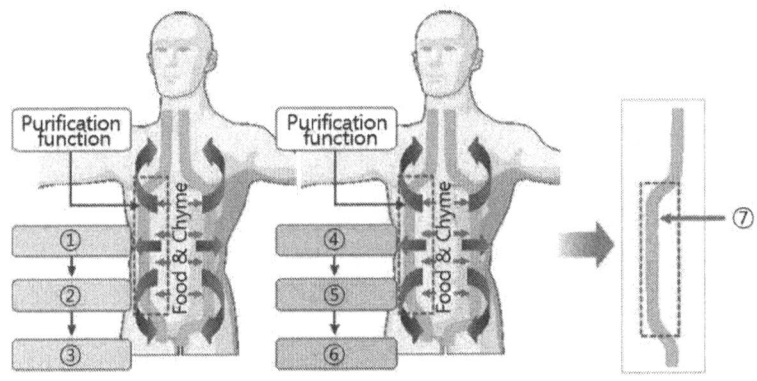

Middle zone Normal state   Middle zone Pollution state

Chyme: semiliquid material which decomposed by gastric digestion of the food.

①Fresh material transmission ②Fresh blood ③Health of whole body ④Dirty material transmission ⑤Dirty blood ⑥Provides problems of whole body ⑦ Middle zone is the front-line of our bodies, so healthy state of this middle zone is very important.

These organs do not function individually but are connected to each other and to cooperate, balance, and check from the point of whole body and perform wholistic digestion, absorption, excretion, immunization, protective guard, and mental functions mysteriously.

The world of stomach is consisted of far more complex and

subtle structure and its functions are too much mysterious that, even with the most highly developed scientific knowledge, its functions cannot be grasped completely, too highly developed for just digesting organs. In fact, it is the first provider of nutrition and at the same time, the septic tank that filters harmful substances from the flowing in enormous amount of materials. Therefore it has to be equipped with right functions. If this became damaged and therefore cannot function well, our body would be flowing with harmful substances through vessels and lymphatic systems. It is like dirty waste would contaminate a whole city if sewerage were overflowed. Our body would slowly fall into the status of illness. The status of this area is a crucial key to proceed to health or to sickness.

TIP 1: Gastrointestinal tract - the front line battle ground

I sometimes toss a question to the gastrointestinal tract disorder patients, 'what are the functions stomach and intestines perform in our body?' Most of them reply, 'they are to digest food', and some add, 'to absorb nutrition.' They are correct, but only half way! To tell it fairly, stomach and intestines are important immune organs. They continuously perform battles to protect from outsiders. Immunization is one of the mysterious functions our body possesses that discerns good or bad for all the flowing-in elements, and resist, tolerate, or fight to keep germs and toxins from spreading over whole body.

How then gastrointestinal tract, the immunizing organs, performs immunization? Its first step is to make the food smallest particles to let them easily absorbed, which is called 'the digestion' process. The stomach physically destroys the food like a mixer does, and with the chemical help of Amylase of saliva, pepsin and acid gastric acid of stomach, the particles become even smaller. Then it passes through small intestine in the form of watery soup. With the help of various digestive enzymes in there, it becomes digested again, absorbed and goes to liver through portal vein. Most of the absorbed foods are used for energy resources and become body elements such as muscles or bones.

Once suspected that poison is contained, immune system of gastrointestinal tract immediately operates, because that harmful substance may damage liver or body. Important thing here is that the immune capacity cannot be too much or too little. If immunization functions weak, the whole body will be tinted with germs and toxins, if too strong, warfare like status will continue. Therefore its immune system must remain highly capable that balances between strength and restraint. With weak immune capacity, it may not remove harmful substances and therefore causes gastrointestinal tract disorder, cirrhosis, arteriosclerosis, migraine, dizziness, diabetes, and various muscle disorders, and those illnesses of which causes are unknown and categorized as 'functional.' On the contrary, too much sensitive immune responses may cause common diseases such as various skin diseases, atopy, rheumatoid arthritis, Behcet's disease, allergy dermatitis, and rhinitis.

As such, gastrointestinal tract is the first gate to discern the coming various foreign objects either harmful or useful, and toil in the front line of the battlefield of body. Gastrointestinal tract is therefore called 'the alert stand guard' for 24 hours to keep the safety of our body in the very front line of battlefield.

TIP 2: The Commander in Chief of the immune system in gastrointestinal tract – Gastrointestinal Tract Lymphoid Tissue (GALT)

There exists an extremely complicated immune system in mucous membrane. The so called GALT (Gut Associated Lymphoid Tissue) plays the front line defense of whole body immunization role. It is the defense system to continuously protect our body from so many kinds of flowing in toxins and foreign objects.

GALT's way of immunization is mysteriously wise. Most immune cells in gastrointestinal tract are programmed to fight unconditionally against foreign objects, and therefore result in certain amount of damages to its own tissues. GALT, however, controls those tissues by considering the whole body in ways they don't harm its own tissues. It leads to wise way of immunization by removing the germs but not receiving any harm from them.

Such way of immunization of GALT is therefore called 'immunological tolerance.'

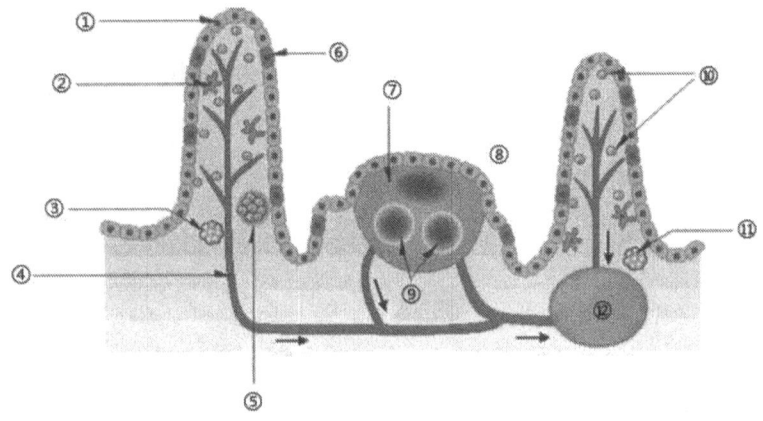

①Intestinal epithelial cell(The cells which divide lumen and intestinal immune system) ②Dendritic cell(The cells which destroy cancer, virus and bacteria) ③Cryptopatch(T cell production) ④Lymphoduct ⑤divided lymphocyte ⑥Endothelial lymphocyte ⑦Peyer's patch(The field of T cell) ⑧Lumen ⑨B lymphocyte ⑩Lymph cell ⑪Cryptopatch ⑫Mesenteric lymph nodes

Suppose two men are fighting. One way of fighting is to violently push and insult each other. The other way is to argue but peacefully solve it in dialogue. The former results in lots of side effects and aftermaths, but the latter will leave no traits of conflicts and come to peaceful solution and prove to be ideal way of response. It has to disarm the toxins of harmful elements without fighting. Therefore immunological tolerance needs wisdom and it is not easy task. The success of such system starts when it does not recognize germs as enemies.

If GALT did not do the immunization that way, our body would continuously suffer from stomachache, diarrhea, vomiting, and infection. The immunological tolerance is a wise system to maintain our body peaceful and to win wars without fighting.

3

Middle zone, hidden treasure in the gastrointestinal tract!

Exterior walls of stomach, though not visible through endoscopy, involve in countless gastrointestinal tract disorders and different kinds of whole body diseases, and functions as septic tank of our body. This research team, after lots of consideration, named it 'Middle Zone.'

Oriental medicine names the digestive system 'Middle Earth.' The function of the stomach and intestine is like earth (soil) which makes all the plants grow on the globe, and absorbs and dissolves many wastes and toxins. Therefore it is compared to 'earth' and it is located in the center of all organs of our body, and therefore we named it 'Middle Earth.' In oriental medicine, it is praised as 'the Middle Earth,' because it underlies the fact that is no less important than brain, and it plays the fundamental role in the center of our body. This concept of digestive system of oriental medicine is no exaggeration, considering the findings of basic science of western medicine on outer walls of mucous membrane. The treasure of 'Middle Earth' lies on outer walls of mucous membrane where endoscopy cannot see but constantly work out enormous amount in the middle zone.

This research team examined lots of terminology to name it with appropriate words. With the idea in oriental medicine that stomach is the center of our body, the concept of 'middle' is taken and to make general audience may call it easy, we decide to name it 'middle zone.'

4

Why is the troubled stomach NOT detected in the endoscopy?

Considering beyond the endoscopy detectable area, the function of the stomach and the extent of gastrointestinal tract disorder is not just about our conventional idea of stomach or diseases on mucous membrane. The middle zone can never be examined unless it is torn apart or see through the abdominal walls, and cannot be seen through endoscopy and therefore medically ignored.

By reading of the endoscopy on the mucous membrane, many diseases on outer walls of mucous membrane have been ignored, and ambiguous names have become the majority of diseases such as functional, neurogenic, and hypersensitive, etc. For those ever increasing digestive cancers such as stomach cancer, colon cancer, and esophageal cancer, accurate medical guidelines and therapies have not been offered and therefore mistakes were made in preparation and treatment of the diseases.

The new stories about gastrointestinal tract have to be quite different from such stories. Not only the endoscopy detectable stomach issues but also issues taking place behind the mucous membrane, the middle zone, we will discuss about gastro-intestinal tract status with far more diverse information.

Gastrointestinal tract – nicknamed '2nd Brain'

'What a stupid guy like food container!'

People call stomach 'food container.' Food container literally means that it holds food. It is partially correct. But 'food container' points to the person of low intelligence and food consuming stupid guy. To sum up, 'food container' simply points to a thoughtless person. But don't you know the following?

The so called, 'food container' is also nicknamed 'the second brain of our body!' Knowing this, we may have to refrain from calling it that way and treat it carefully with respect.

Imagine now that we go to a fitness center to exercise. Finishing up the warming up exercise, in order to make up the muscular look, we are about to do the dumbbell. Our brain will run swiftly like a computer circuit does. Brain nerves of various areas discuss about the best way to lift it, and the frontal lobe discerns the final result, and gives command to motor nerves. The motor nerves then send out signals to muscles to move. Muscles then contract to move the hard bones to lift the dumbbell. The whole process is performed by 'I' (brain) that discerns and controls to make it happen. This is called 'voluntary movement.' But heart or stomach and intestines are not the organs that I can command to do this or that. It is done by involuntary ways of movement system. These nerves that are controlled by themselves is called 'autonomic nerve.'

The splanchnic nerve in the gastrointestinal tract is automatic nerve. It automatically discerns and controls on almost all the situations happening in stomach and intestines. There is external nervous system in stomach and intestines, and it delivers information from splanchnic nerve to brain and spinal cord to cooperate with each other, but most of the cases, it discerns by itself and perform without interference of brain. It is like front desk clerks voluntarily discern and execute issues without acquiring approval from CEO.

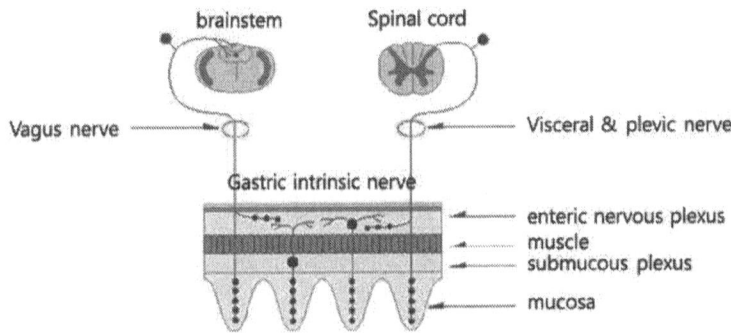

This autonomic splanchnic nerve in the stomach and intestines perform far more important roles than any other organs. It has the most number of nerves next only to brain, and has five times more nerves than the spinal nerve, the nerve specialized organ. Why does it need this many nerves?

This is probably because of the urgent need of discerning and handling so many kinds of foods that are coming continuously from outside. Splanchnic nerve sorts out foods from outside to good ingredients and poisonous ones and put all those sorted out information to splanchnic nerves and immune cells in the gastrointestinal tract. Furthermore, based on the remembered information, nervous system and immune system properly handle the foods according to the contents by cooperating with each other. Its process of cooperating is very complex and sophisticated. Though receiving a little bit of interference from brain, most of the time the two get united and solve the issues. As we can see, gastrointestinal tract is pretty smart organ in discerning and operating by itself to protect and maintain our body. This is the reason why it is nicknamed 'the second brain' and receives special recognition.

TIP: The embarrassing 'burp and fart'

Burp is the gas that escapes through mouth, and fart is the one through anus. Gas is produced in gastrointestinal tract when eating or drinking food, when breathing in air is taken to stomach, and when food fermented and decomposed by germs. Our body physiologically urged to let the gas out of body. The main pathological reason is that the eaten food, being not properly digested and absorbed, go down to intestines in chyme and feed the germs existing there, and various gases are made. Without these reasons, burp and fart can be still habitual. It is when sphincter muscle from esophageal to stomach weakened or smooth muscle in the middle zone hardened, and gas cannot go down further but reflux. Especially when sphincter muscles become weakened, we don't feel the sense of food going down smoothly, and that cause us to burp intentionally. When repeated, it becomes worse and develops to habitual burping. In oriental medicine, when stomach becomes badly weakened, eaten food does not go down the tract but reflux. It is therefore called 'regurgitation,' or 'frequent vomiting.'

Part 04

True Nature of Gastrointestinal Tract Disorder Unveiled

1
Indigestion, obvious symptoms but no reasons?

Among gastrointestinal tract disorders, some disorders are detectable through endoscopy and microscope such as, gastritis, gastric ulcer, polyp, and stomach cancer. But there are more disorders that are not visible on endoscopy or microscope but come with symptoms of burp, bloating, indigestion, uncomfortable stomach with headache, pain, and heartburn. There is no smoke without fire! There are clear causes to functional gastrointestinal tract disorders. Lots of researches have strived to find the causes but failed to grasp the exact reality of them. Some researchers use the term 'inflammation' again and claim that it is because of micro inflammation. In recent years, pace maker that is cajal cell of gastrointestinal muscle movements seems to be involved in the cause of the disorders, some claim.

The many unanswered symptoms of gastrointestinal disorders appear because of the destructions of immune organs, nerves, secretory organs such as neurohormone and enzyme, locomotive organs such as muscles and vessels in the middle zone. How then the middle zone becomes destructed?

Greatest accident in the body: Mucous membrane becomes degenerated!

2

Guard of our body, Mucous membrane gate!

The surface of mucous membrane of stomach and intestines looks pink colored and folded, and looks shiny because of the gastric juice on it. When zooming in the mucous membrane tissues, cells are closely meshed together like fingers are well meshed when our hands are folded together.

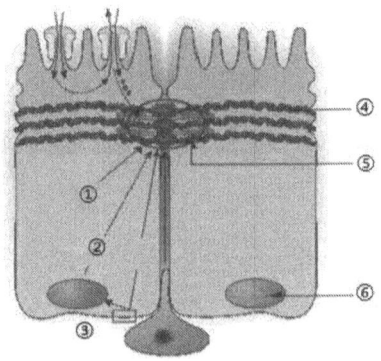

Dense connection structure of gastric mucous cells

①Dense connection ②Concerning on opening and closing of dense connection ③ Cytokine ④Dense connection control ring(actin, myosin) ⑤Protein structure connecting between mucous cells(material transmission gate) ⑥Nucleus

Amazing thing is that there are gates in between the meshed tissues, and the gates repeat opening and closing like the check point at the airport, opening up when passing the inspection, closing when problems arise. These gates are closed and stop the harmful toxins or not yet dissolved high molecular substances from entering in. The gates are open when well-dissolved substances are present. They are to be delivered to whole body through liver. When the meshed up tissues are damaged for some reasons, the gates still open at the presence of harmful substances.

The meshed up tissues abnormally open when mucous membrane become degenerated by infecting substances, germs, toxins from food wastes, alcohols, chemicals, drugs, Helicobacter, degeneration of cytokine that controls immune cells in the gastrointestinal tract.

3

Cause of mucous membrane damage - Everything!

If mucous membrane damaged, middle zone collapses!

The mucous membrane being degenerated is no little accident for our body. When mucous membrane broke, harmful or undissolved high molecular substances that should not be allowed to enter, may still come to the middle zone. If the zone gets polluted by harmful substances, different kinds of problems arise in the gastrointestinal tract such as immune disorder against food, nervous reactions disorders, and motor disturbances. This polluted status of the middle zone will spread over the whole body through blood vessels and lymphatic system and become the breeding ground of lots of diseases.

For these reasons, protecting mucous membrane is a crucial premise for keeping our health. However, we tend to carelessly treat mucous membrane in our diet without understanding the importance of the mucous membrane.

Next, we want to consider the causes of mucous membrane damages. It is as diverse as the complex stomach and intestines issues. It lists all the possible causes that may prompt mucous membrane problems including wrong eating habits such as eating fast, eating heavy, and overeating. These reasons may eventually damage our stomach and intestines and can cause cancers, diabetes, strokes, skin troubles, and the whole body diseases.

Cause of mucous membrane damage – everything!

* Pathogenic microorganism and infiltration of germs
* Toxins from eating fast, eating heavy, and overeating
* Stress
* Chemicals and polluted substances Alcohols
* Excessive increase of mastocyte, the active cells of gastro-intestinal tract
* Helicobacter
* Active oxygen
* Gastrointestinal function decrease
* Other diseases such as diabetes or heart disease
* Pathological degeneration of cytokine

Pathogenic microorganism and infiltration of germs

E. Coli or food poisoning bacteria that cause problems in summer easily stick to gastrointestinal tract walls and produce toxins, damage mucous membrane, and destroy various kinds of enzymes. Typical example is that they destroy bile and protein-digesting enzymes secreted from pancreas and lower the digestion and absorption of fat and protein. Toxins of microorganism and germs also penetrate epithelial cells of gastrointestinal tract and cause diseases such as diarrhea, fever, stomachache, and may develop to blood poisoning.

Toxins from bingeing, overeating, irregular overeating

Overeating, irregular overeating, bingeing, vomiting, and reflux inflict direct damages to mucous membrane and muscles of gastrointestinal tract and produce undissolved wastes and therefore create environments where germs can grow well. Since digestive enzymes work mostly on the surface of food, this way of eating cause the chunk of food go down the stomach and remained undissolved there. The undissolved foods, germs increased with the food, and the poisons eventually damage the mucous membrane of the gastrointestinal tract and pollute the middle zone.

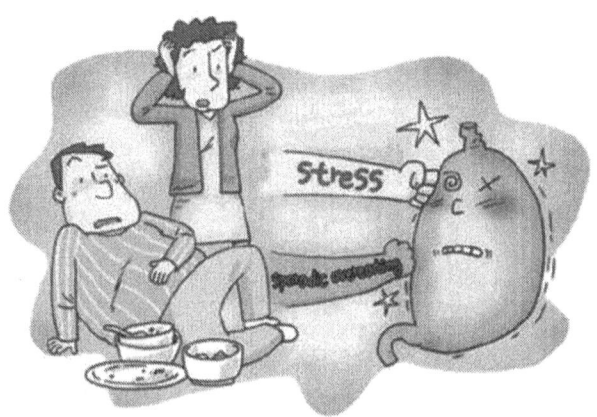

<Stop here! >

Why do abnormal bacteria grow inside?

Pathogenic bacteria grow inside the gastrointestinal tract in the following conditions. Autonomic nervous diseases such as diabetic neuropathy, intestinal movements disorder by excessive sugar intake, gastric acid decrease in the tract, prolonged intake of gastric acid restrainers, bile secreting decrease, pancreas enzyme decrease, overeating, irregular overeating, bingeing, and food wastes caused by polluted substances creates suitable environment for bacteria increase inside.

Functions of normal bacteria!

Normal bacteria restrain the increase of harmful bacteria in our body and produces anti-bacteria substance that can fight back the germs. Besides this, it helps the growth and activities of microvilli, creating components of intestinal muscles, playing important role in forming the walls of intestinal tube, removing poisonous substance, stimulating immune system in gastro-intestinal tract and the like positive roles.

Getting angry means direct hit to gastrointestinal tract – Stressed out

Most of the stress we receive influence pituitary gland and it in return stimulates adrenal cortex to cause it secrete stress hormones. According to the experiments on mice, stress hormones break up the meshed tissues of intestines, and let the high molecular food particles penetrate. It also increases the number of mastocyte of mucous membrane and causes to release excessive gastric acid, and to cause gastrointestinal troubles such as infection, heartburn, and pain.

Stress caused gastrointestinal disorder mechanism
- ☞ Stress → adrenal cortex hormones → stimulates mastocyte → promotes secreting histamine → releases gastric acid → mucous membrane damage
- ☞ Stress → abnormal increase of bacteria inside the gastrointestinal tract → with damaged mucous membrane, more penetrate the middle zone

Eaten chemical drugs or polluted substances

Eating too much food additives such as preservatives, pesticide, MSG, bleach, or agricultural chemicals, beyond the capacity of mucous membrane defense mechanism, one may experience immediate mucous membrane damage and gastrointestinal tract disorders. After taking anti-inflammatory drugs or antibiotics, one may experience gastroenteritis. It also means the chemical drugs have damaged mucous membrane.

Drinking alcohols

Alcohols can damage mucous membrane more than any other

foods do. It makes alcohol and poison transfer to liver fast. Too much alcohol directly stimulates the mucous membrane to cause gastroenteritis and therefore diarrhea and stomachache may follow. Gastrointestinal tract disorders happen more often to chronic alcohol drinkers. It is not because of the direct stimulation of alcohol but rather because of the continuous intake, metabolic and detoxicating functions of the liver become damaged and too much nitric oxide are produced and therefore gastrointestinal tract disorder develop.

Excessive increase of mastocyte makes it worse

Mastocyte is on our skin and around blood vessels and mucous membrane of gastrointestinal tract and functions as secreting good mucus to mucous membrane, controlling of blood flow and movement of stomach and intestines, activating immune response, and forming blood vessels. It then raises low blood pressures, controls permeability of mucus cells and promote absorbability, activate immune response, prevent blood clotting, and do other important positive functions. If it is too many, it damages the gastrointestinal tract.

Mastocyte, in order to perform the above described functions, makes use of histamine or heparin, if number of mastocyte increases because of stress or food allergy or inflammatory intestinal diseases, histamine substance is also produced excessively and immune response become too sensitive and therefore various intestinal diseases appear. It also damages the meshed tissues of the mucous membrane, and poisonous substance that have infiltrated through outer walls of mucous membrane causes the whole body diseases.

It is known that the number of mastocyte becomes increased by stresses such as anger, or poisons or stimulating foods. In the process of stresses, poisons, stimulating foods damaging gastrointestinal tract, mastocyte is somehow connected, we know.

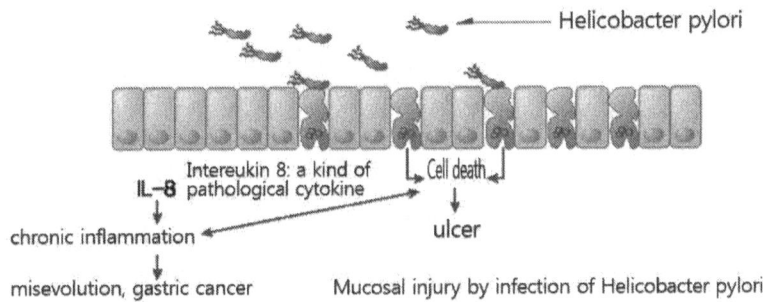

Mucosal injury by infection of Helicobacter pylori

Helicobacter!

Epithelial cells of stomach mucous membrane maintains balances by continuously manufacturing, multiplying, and perishing, But once infected by helicobacter, its cycle of growth and death becomes too fast, Overall health of mucous membrane then becomes worse and aging process accelerating. Once mucous membrane becomes weakened and aging, it paves the road to chronic inflammation, forming ulcers, and developing gastric cancer.

Active oxygen – poison of all diseases

The oxygen we breathe is the essential element in producing energy of our body. However, when metabolic process is not stable and oxygen is not treated, excessive oxygen appears. It is called active oxygen. This oxidizes our body and does, for the most part, harmful function. Oxidation is the same natural process as steel becomes rusty. As active oxygen makes steel rusty, it also attack and change the function of cell membrane, cell contents and gene. Eventually protein-producing function decreases, mutation of gene takes place, and gives cause for different kinds of disease.

Mucous membrane gets destroyed with the influence of helicobacter or salted preserve food, and active oxygen is involved in this process. The proof is that by taking drugs to restrain active oxygen, gastritis and gastric cancer case reduced. Active oxygen is produced by ischemic damage or inflammatory intestine disorders, non-steroidal painkiller, and ethanol. Recently, active oxygen is to be seen as the source of destroying mucous membrane as in different kinds of intestine mucous disorders such as gastric ulcer and colitis.

When gastrointestinal tract becomes weak

Damage caused by blood supply disorder in the gastrointestinal tract

Blood is supplied to heart and kidney first and then to gastrointestinal tract. Therefore ischemia often happens. Once a little stressed, one may feel stomachache and indigestion. People who get easily stressed and suffer from weak heart tend to have bad blood supply to gastrointestinal tract. In this case, deficient supply of oxygen to gastrointestinal tract and lowered mucus regeneration capacity create infection cause substances. It then cause lots of gastrointestinal tract disorder.

People born with weak gastrointestinal tract capacity or with myasthenia

Having weak gastrointestinal tract can mean the following: Immune function of gastrointestinal tract decreased, gastric acid reduced, or gastrointestinal muscle motility lowered.

If Immune function decreased and gastric acid reduced, a little bit of spicy food or small amount of poison contained food can cause infection or different kinds of indigestion. Once gastrointestinal muscle motility decreased, it is hard to make the food go down the tract, and therefore make the stomach upset often, stuffy pit of the stomach, reflux, gas bloating, or dyschezia (hard to make bowel movement). When blood supply is not properly done, a little of bit stress may cause ischemia and therefore often have gastrointestinal disorders such as feeling stomachache or inflammation. When mucus of the mucous membrane reduces, ulcer related diseases happen because of the gastric acid attack. Spicy foods or poisons can cause mucous membrane damage.

Other diseases that cause mucous membrane disorder

Metabolic diseases such as diabetes and heart diseases, for example, heart failures, influence gastrointestinal tract issues. Especially when one suffers diabetes more than 10 years, micro blood vessels bring nerve damage and it then may cause lots of gastrointestinal tract disorder and whole body disorder symptoms. If micro blood vessels damaged, gastrointestinal tract mucus cannot be produced easily and blood supply becomes difficult and that may trigger stomach mucous membrane damage and indigestion disorders. Then it shows similar symptoms as myasthenia or hypersensitive intestine disorders. When nerve damage progresses, alarm function of nerves decreases and lots of poisons permeate to the whole body through outer walls of the gastrointestinal tract. It may trigger whole body diseases such as arteriosclerosis, cirrhosis, renal failure, angina, joint diseases, and gout.

Pathological degeneration of Cytokine - the information delivery agent in gastrointestinal tract!

In order to efficiently carry out the immune response, it should not unconditionally fight back the bacteria or poison that are coming from outside. If the response were always like at war, our body would not get away from inflammation. Real immune should not wreak havoc in our body just to get rid of bad elements that have intruded. To do this, various immune cells closely cooperate and choose highly developed immune formats.

In order to react best to bacteria and harmful poisons, immune cells have to deliver the information with each other for accomplishing normal immune capacity. Such activity of information sharing and communication is done by cytokine. Cytokine functions like a messenger in military. It forms highly efficient frontline among immune cells. When, however, cytokine becomes pathologically degenerated for some reasons, wrong information is delivered among immune cells and abnormal immune procedures are carried out and cause lots of middle zone problems, gastrointestinal disorders, and autoimmune disorders.

Pathological cytokine is produced chiefly in the process of immune response to poisonous foods and by the side effect of stress.

<Stop here!>

Cytokine was discovered in the process of a research in 1950s throughout 1970 to find out what kinds of proteins involve in immune response to antigen or to infectious diseases. Interferon, the first physiological cytokine, has been proved to restrain virus infection. IL-1 (Inteorukin), the typical pathological cytokine, is revealed to cause heating as a pyrogen in various infectious diseases.

TIP: Gastrointestinal noise - water sound

When feeling hungry, we hear noise in the belly. It is for the stomach to cry for the food. When it is time to eat, stomach and intestines get ready for receiving food. The noise at this time will disappear upon eating. When not mealtime, but still hear the sound, it is when stomach and intestines make too much movements. Vermicular movements are for intestines to make continuous movements from esophagus toward anus. Strong vermicular movements means that it tries to make the food residues get out of the body. In other words, intestines feel that the food residues make troubles. It is when food contains poisons or when over-eating leaves the chime, and intestines carries out extra vermicular movements to let it move, and it produces sounds in the process. In many occasions, however, intestines become sensitive because of small inflammatory changes. If it does not cause pain or diarrhea and does not influence daily activities, it does not matter much. But it is better to find out the cause of being sensitive. Sometimes it becomes full of gas and makes noise all the time. It is because not enough moisture get absorbed in the large intestine and moisture undercurrent is formed in the intestines. Oriental medicine explains that it lacks yang energy. If intestines become cold, it is difficult to absorb water.

4

Middle zone damage leads to hardening of outer wall of gastrointestinal tract

When defense mechanism of mucous membrane gets degenerated, middle zone becomes damaged and new forms of gastrointestinal tract and whole body diseases start. This has been undetectable by endoscopy.

When Weedahm Oriental Hospital conducted a clinical research in 2003, those patients who had been categorized with neurogenic, functional gastrointestinal tract disorders had something in common; outer walls of their stomach and intestines got swollen and hardened. I did not have scientific understanding of why outer walls of the mucous membrane should swell and harden, because I had no medical understanding of middle zone and its pathological status at the time. But I now grasp the reality as it has been unveiled.

True nature of potbelly

In public bathhouses, people with their lower abdomen significantly protruded are sighted. We commonly call this 'potbelly' and think it may because of excessive belly fat. Is it only because of belly fat? When pressing down the belly of these people, we feel the hardened part of it, and most of them complain severe pain. If it is only fat, it can't be painful. If it is hardened and feeling painful when pressed down, it must be the area where blood vessels and nerves spread.

We can guess that this is the middle zone where blood vessels, nerves, muscles of outer walls of stomach and intestines exist. Therefore, some parts of potbelly, physically protruding, are the hardened and swollen part of middle zone of outer walls of stomach and intestines. We cannot dismiss the potbelly as the sign of 'maturity' anymore. We may have to realize that a severe form of disease lies inside there.

Stomach and intestines get intramuscular pain

What does it mean to have stomach and intestines hardened and swollen? We may understand it with ease by examining organs existing in the middle zone.

The outer walls of stomach and intestines are muscle tissues, and the smooth muscle becomes swollen and hardened. When shoulders or nape of neck become stiff, hardened, and painful, we call it 'I get dahm' in Korean. The English translation of it can be 'get intramuscular pain.' As such, stomach and intestines can also get intramuscular pain. It may become stony hardened, feeling painful when pressed, its motility decreased, and digestion and excretion become difficult.

Lymph nodes, the main immune organ, may have swollen. Lymph nodes may have edema caused by poisons, bacteria, and wastes. If the problem continues, it becomes hardened.

In stomach and intestines, many blood vessels form structures and blood is supplied through them. But stress caused ischemia, wastes caused narrow blood vessels, and extravagated blood remaining in the vessels may interfere the blood flow in the vessels and muscle tissues may become even more hardened.

With these complex changes, outer walls of stomach and intestines become hardened by and large, swelling up in shapes, and its inside organs, such as muscles, immune cells, nerves, and blood vessels decline in function or pathological condition progress such as stopping or degenerating in function.

When palpating on the abdomen, we can feel hardened and swollen tissues. When pressed, they will complain pain. We call this overall status 'get Dahm (intramuscular pain).'

As such, when Dahm (intramuscular pain) is formed in gastrointestinal tract, various problems arise; abnormal immune system and nerve response, harmful substance permeability increase that cause to accumulate poisons, and change of Cajal cell (the motility controlling cell). Therefore the Dahm disease (intramuscular pain) is the essence of gastrointestinal tract disorders we suffer usually.

What is 'Dahm disease' (intramuscular pain) that oriental medicine talks?

The term 'Dahm' is the combination of the word 'inflammation' and the word 'disease.' The reason why Dahm is based on the word 'inflammation' is as following. Though it is not an inflammation in itself, its root is from inflammation, and when the inflammation lasts long, it proceeds to Dahm, the intramuscular pain. Inflammation is a kind of symptoms or phenomena. But Dahm is a disease in deeper dimension. It is not a temporary symptom that was here but disappears next moment. It is already degenerated and do not operate properly or it may become breeding bed of other diseases. Inflammation becomes Dahm disease as described in the following.

In the process of immune response to various elements, inflammation takes place along with heat in histiocyte. The inflammation is to return to its original status according to the constancy mechanism. If it is re-infected in the meantime, or poisonous environment becomes aggravated by ways of fatigue, stress, excessive alcohol, inflammation is not healed but proceeds to worse status. Like this, histiocyte becomes degenerated beyond the status of inflammation. It is called Dahm disease.

Dahm disease appears differently depending on its location. If Dahm is accumulated in the gastrointestinal muscles systems, its muscles swell up and hardened. Then it causes motor disturbance of gastrointestinal muscle and pain, and therefore cannot make food go down the tract or gastrospasm often happens. Cajal cells, the motility controlling cell, disappear and therefore stomach activities significantly reduced, and multiplication of gastrointestinal tissues may progress.

If Dahm is accumulated in the gastrointestinal immune systems, it cannot restrain germs and cannot remove harmful elements on time, and therefore its environment inside becomes dirty.

If Dahm is accumulated in nervous systems, its alarm system cannot work when harmful elements should invade, and many poisonous diseases may spread all over the body, and it can conversely become too sensitive to normal substances that diarrhea, stomachache, vomiting, and infection may appear.

5

Gastrointestinal tract disorder that has symptoms but no causes: 'Phlegm Mass Disorder'

When liver hardened, 'Cirrhosis,' how about gastrointestinal tract hardened?

When finding the causes of gastrointestinal tract disorder, this research team decided to name the new disease, because it is different from the mucous disease such as gastritis or gastric ulcer that are caused by mucous membrane damage inside the stomach and intestines. After some time of consideration, we named it 'Phlegm Mass Disorder.' The disease starts with the middle zone when polluted by food wastes or poisons, and undergo chemical changes and the tissues become hardened and swelled up and its shape changed. We combined the word 'Phlegm (Dahm) to mean waste or poison and 'Mass (Juk)' and finally call it 'Phlegm Mass Disorder.'

6

The reality of Phlegm Mass Disorder

Habitual fast eating, overeating or sporadic heavy eating makes the food not dissolved completely in the gastrointestinal tract, and leave chyme like food waste in the tract. These waste flow the tract and produce lots of poisons. When eating poison containing foods such as chemicals, preservatives, pesticide, and heavy metals, the poisons damage the mucous membrane of stomach and intestines and make epithelial barrier broken. Through the degenerated mucous membrane cells, the contents in high molecule and poisons start permeating and harmful substances slowly accumulated on immune cells, outer wall muscle layer, blood vessel system and lymphatic systems and mucous membrane outer wall tissue become swell up and hardened.

As mucous membrane of gastrointestinal tract gets deteriorated by food wastes, poisons, and harmful substances, various organs such as immune organs, nervous systems, nervous hormone systems, muscle, and blood vessel systems are damaged and middle zone in general becomes hardened and swells up, it is called Phlegm Mass Disorder. Following is how each organ of middle zone actually degenerated by Phlegm Mass Disorder and their symptoms.

Pathological mechanism	Middle zone damage & degeneration	Phlegm Mass Disorder
* mucous membrane damage * epithelial cells damage * harmful substance permeability rating increase * harmful substance basal cells approaching	* lymphatic systems edema & damage * blood circulation disorder & blood vessels degeneration * Cajal cell extinction or inactivation causes muscle hardening & motility disorder	* outer walls of stomach and intestines thickening & hardening

Immune system disorder

When epithelial barrier is broken, the contents inside of intestines and harmful substances approach the immune cells and damage the immune system and cause the system to respond with abnormal immune response. Once damaged in the immune system, various kinds of diseases may appear such as gastritis, enteritis, Crohn disease, various autoimmune disease, dermatopathy, and joint disease.

Nervous system damage

To protect our body, epithelial cells or immune cells on the mucous membrane layers deal with poisons, foreign high molecular substance, and pathogenic bacteria that are entering gastrointestinal tract.

In cooperation with brain, on the scale of whole body, the cells control the energy and moisture level so as not to become too much or too little. When eating too much, therefore, they cause the sense of bloating, vomiting, or diarrhea; or when eating little, they cause sense of hunger and thirsty and make the body supplement them. The cells, to defend gastrointestinal tract, also produce the sense of pain and uncomfortableness against poisons, harmful substances, or other physical, chemical stimulating elements. All these responses are physiological and normal response to protect the body, and we cannot consciously feel it, because it is performed by autonomic nervous system.

For various reasons when nerves get damaged, the cells react too sensitively to normal food or to a little bit of stress and cause to feel pain, convulsion, and abnormal bowel movements.

In the process of immune response to various poisons and harmful foods, a pathological medium is isolated, so called 'pathological cytokine' and it causes unnecessary sensitive responses. Nervous system can be also degenerated by food wastes or poison pollution. Once nervous system gets degenerated, alarm function of gastrointestinal tract gets impaired and sends out wrong information to brain and body protection mechanism begins to degenerate. For example, though overeating, sporadic overeating, or taking harmful foods continually, cells may not question the issue and not send out alarm message to brain, and feel that digestion goes on well and not feeling pain. Though having eaten to the full, body feels like to eat more, and feeling abnormal urge to eat something before going to bed.

On the surface, one may feel digestion goes on well, but it may result in significant cases of gastric cancer, colon cancer, stroke, diabetes, arteriosclerosis, cirrhosis, skin diseases, gout, arthritis, headache, and dizziness.

Nervous system degeneration may cause interesting phenomenon. When eating same food only, our body may codify the food and store it inside and create the nervous response to favor the food only. Kids of nowadays prefer and insist on eating instant foods, fast foods or pizza, those rather harmful foods, then become addicted to eat the food because of the mechanism of the body.

When gastrointestinal tract alarm system gets impaired, eating meal fast or eating too much or eating poison containing foods does not give any uncomfortable symptoms. Rather one may feel like eating more. This is because alarm function of the splanchnic nerves gets impaired, not because the gastrointestinal tract is strong. In the meantime, the middle zone of outer walls of gastrointestinal tract get significantly damaged by food poisons. On the surface level, one may think that digestion goes well, but in reality, it starts conceiving big diseases such as gastric cancer colon cancer, stroke, diabetes, arteriosclerosis, cirrhosis, skin diseases, arthritis, gout, and dizziness. As such, alarm system damage may cause whole body diseases. In actuality, those hospitalized stoke, diabetes, and arthritis patients usually used to eat well, overeat and think that their stomach could digest even stones. Why were these people so confident of their health but now lie in hospital beds with serious illness? The reason is that they have eaten recklessly, thinking that they digest everything well when in reality their alarm system inside got broken.

We now have to realize the importance of alarm system. Know that stomach and intestines say something when we have gastrointestinal tract symptoms such as bloating, pain, vomit, and diarrhea. These symptoms are very important for our body. It is to say stop eating there, to say that we better be careful because it is dangerous food, to inform us, the owner of the stomach.

The alarm system of gastrointestinal tract gets broken because eating fast, overeating, sporadic overeating, and poisonous food causes poisons get accumulated on splanchnic nerves of gastrointestinal tract, and its nerves get degenerated. Once the nerves get degenerated, it does not discern good or bad on foods and sends out unconditional OK sign to all foods, and worse yet, favoring the bad foods. Nowadays when kids get used to instant foods or fast foods, they favor those foods. It shows how excessive intake of specific foods and its poisons degenerate nerves.

Nervous hormones' excess response

Nervous hormone secreting cells of gastrointestinal tract functions as taste bud of tongue and provides the sensory nerves of mucous membrane epithelial cells with information on substances that have come to stomach and intestines to deal with harmful or damaging elements.

For example, epithelial cells of mucous membrane can get

damaged because of physical forces, alcohols, painkillers, spicy foods, and bile reflux. Once epithelial cells get damaged, pepsin, the hydrochloric acid and protein digesting enzyme, becomes radically aggressive agent and stomach tissues become destroyed. When stomach tissues destroyed, nervous hormones and exogenous nerves immediately stimulate brain and spinal chord to run defense system, such as increasing blood flow, to protect stomach and intestines.

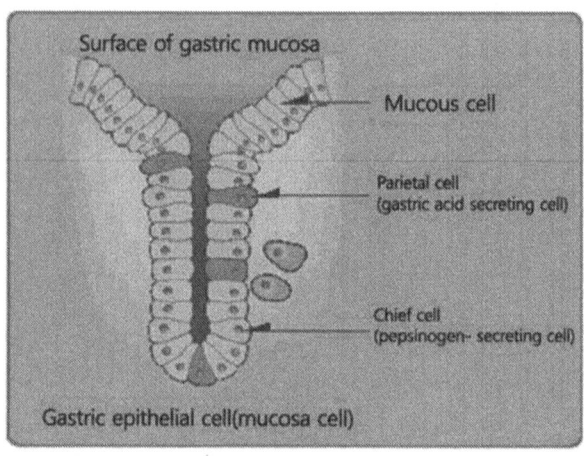

However, if infection, inflammation, or damages continue to happen, nerve hormones or sensory nerves undergo severe functional change. Once functions damaged, even though causative agent should disappear, its symptoms would remain. This pathological change of nerve hormones and sensory system make excessive response to substances that are flowing to gastrointestinal tract, and deliver sensitive and distorted information to brain and cause us to feel pain, heartburn, diarrhea, and nausea. When we feel that our stomach and intestines become sensitive, it is because there are problems in these nerve hormones and sensory system, and furthermore, there is change in brain's central dealing system.

Gastrointestinal tract muscle issues

Vermicular movements and mixing work of gastrointestinal tract is done by smooth muscles. Strong smooth muscles guarantee the smooth digestion and bowel movements.

If smooth muscles get hardened, motility capacity of gastrointestinal tract decreased and various symptoms appear such as stuffed feeling on pit of the stomach, filling of gas, reflux, burp, dyschezia (hard to make bowel movement), and frequent stomach upset. The cause of smooth muscle becoming hardened has not been known in the medical circle. Cajal cells are discovered recently, however, which is known as the pace maker of smooth muscle movements, and the decrease of number of Cajal cells leads to the lowered motility of gastrointestinal tract movements. How the number of Cajal cells reduced is not known yet. But when patients with severe gastrointestinal motility disorder are treated with phlegm mass disorder treatment and their hardened outer walls of gastrointestinal tract relieved, digest movements recovered. Therefore it is considered that reduction of number of Cajal cells has something to do with Phlegm Mass poison in the gastrointestinal tract.

Relationship between phlegm mass disorder, Cajal cells, and gastrointestinal tract movement!

The phenomenon of outer walls of gastrointestinal tract swelling up and hardening was confirmed in 2006 with the tester that had been designed to examine the organs. Most of the patients whose outer walls of the gastrointestinal tract swelled up and hardened commonly experienced gastrointestinal tract motility decrease. In this patient group, such symptoms are observed as cirrhosis, diabetes, uterine myoma, prostate syndrome, breast node, frequent kidney diseases, and myalgia. These clinical phenomena have something to do with outer walls of stomach and intestines, i.e., smooth muscle's swelling up and hardening and tissue multiplication around the area Cajal cells spread, we can infer.

Blood circulation disorder in gastrointestinal tract

Blood circulation is essential element in performing physiological functions such as gastrointestinal tract movements, immune, and nerve response. It also becomes the recovering agent when these functions get damaged. When blood circulation goes on well, damaged organs can get easily repaired.

There are different kinds of blood circulation disorders; blood supply itself is not enough, viscosity of blood is too high to circulate (murky or sticky blood), and blood vessel narrowed. They are medically called, ischemia, extravasated blood, respectively. Ischemia happens when heart functions weak or blood supply becoming not sufficient because of stress. Extravasated blood happens as the result of bleeding or aftermath of it, the impure blood leaves blood clot on the blood vessel walls and impedes the blood circulation.

Ischemia leads to damage of gastrointestinal tract mucous membrane and susceptible to damage. Endotoxin environment is formed, and blood flow can be reversed, and the toxin spread to other organs, it then causes autoimmune disease such as cardiac infarction and Behcet's disease. It causes inflammation agents to take place often, oxygen supply to stomach and intestines decreased, and mucous membrane restoration capacity lowered.

Especially when phlegm mass settles down in blood vessels, its walls get hardened or narrowed, and promotes phlegm mass poisons, and forms the basis of chronic or acute stomach disorders. It also supplies the murky and polluted blood to liver and therefore causes many a whole body disorders.

TIP: The most frequent disorder, 'Gastritis'

Gastritis is a symptom that has inflammation in the stomach. In Chinese characters, of the word, 'Inflammation' signifies a symptom that has 'flame.' In English, it also has 'flame' in the letter. When inflammation happens, it has fever, swelling, pain, and redness in that area. The stomach becomes so called, 'red and sore.' On endoscopy, gastritis is confirmed with the presence of color change, discharge, and edema. With biopsy, closer examination of inflamed cells, tissue changes, and the presence of Helicobacter. In western medicine, Inflammation causes 90% of all diseases.

Inflammation itself is not a disease. It is a phenomenon caused by a disease. It is the result of a defense by a living tissue to a certain stimulus such as germs or toxins. When an inflammation is diagnosed, it is to confirm the presence of surface problem. To treat inflammation is to treat phenomena, not the disease itself. Beneath the surfaced 'inflammation,' disorders take place to immune system, nervous system, muscle, various agent substances, and vascular system, and cause sensitive immune and nervous response, harmful substance inflow by permeability increase, nervous endocrine control disorder, and the motility control cell – Cajal cells change. This is the nature of gastrointestinal tract disorder.

(Gastrointestinal tract security/alarm system is more sophisticated than ADT system)

To see how splanchnic nerves of gastrointestinal tract deals with the harmful substances coming from outside is very interesting and insightful. To protect our body, splanchnic nerves along with exogenous nerves run alarm system. Its system is equipped with very much sophisticated and various channels.

1. First stage alarm: 'poison, high molecular substance, pathological germs infiltrated!'
Epithelial cells and immune cells on mucous membrane layers, secreting cells inside the intestines detect and respond!
2. Second stage alarm: 'Roger!'
Endogenous nerves receive information from epithelial nerves and immune alarm system.
3. Third stage alarm: 'It start feeling pain.'
Monitoring the information, it delivers to brain through exogenous nerves.

It sends messages to brain to say that 'Harmful substance has entered, or too much food has come, and it is most likely that poison would spread to whole body, therefore create symptoms such as pain, vomiting, bloating, and diarrhea.'

There is a well-developed nervous system in gastrointestinal tract. It is to examine whether too much food has come inside, poison is contained, or by eating hastily non-digestible high molecular substances are contained. It stands guard against poisons spread over the body that are derived from wrong way of eating. The way of protecting body is done, with the help of brain, by making various gastrointestinal symptoms such as upset stomach, vomit, pain, and diarrhea. Splanchnic nervous system of gastrointestinal tract discerns the issue and informs brain to activate the symptoms.

(Cajal Cells)

Cajal cells were discovered by Cajal in 1911. They exist between gastrointestinal nerve system and smooth muscle and function as pace maker of autonomic movements. Cajal cells are controlled by serotonin, the emotion control nervous substance. It is because of this reason that we digest well when feeling good and not well when feeling gloomy or stressed. Gastrointestinal tract movements are done by nerves and by muscles. Movements done by nerves are controlled by various nerve carrier substances and hormones, and those done by muscles are controlled mostly by Cajal cells.

Researches on Cajal cells reduction caused diseases

The number of Cajal cells is significantly reduced in the following patients; constipation patients caused by Intestine motility declining, acquired mega-colon patients, and gastrointestinal tract benign tumor (epilepsy tissue tumor, GISTs). It reports the fact that reduction of Cajal cells has something to do with smooth muscle's motility declining and tissue multiplication.

In addition to this, prostatism, breast line tissue multiplication, and bladder contractile strength declining took place where Cajal cells are spread in such places as prostate, breast, and kidney. In these diseases, Cajal cell declining commonly took place. It again points out that Cajal cells are directly involved in tissue multiplication and smooth muscle movements. It is revealed that Cajal cells exist in exocrine gland of pancreas, liver portal vein, and celiac artery. It is therefore expected that *diabetes, cirrhosis, and arteriosclerosis are also relevant to Cajal cells. Only if we can find out scientifically why Cajal cells become reduced, above mentioned diseases may find ways to healing.*

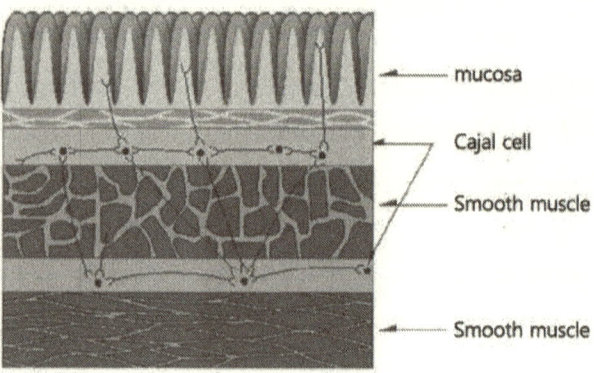

General way of addressing Cajal cells is 'Interstitial Cell of Cajal,' or ICC in short. It is because most of them are in gastrointestinal tract muscle layers, ICC-IM (Interstitial Cell of Cajal intramuscular.) It is relevant to the phlegm mass disorder symptoms, I believe, considering the function of it and accompanying diseases when it decreased in numbers.

Interesting thing is that when phlegm poison removal and blood circulation improving medication was prescribed, the hardened and swollen part of the outer walls of stomach and intestines became relieved soft and we witnessed the reliving of problems of diabetes, cirrhosis, bladder diseases, and uterine myoma, not to speak of gastrointestinal disorders.

There should be animal testing later, where phlegm mass disorder artificially put on, checking Cajal cells activity index and number of cells decrease, and conduct research on how phlegm mass poisons affect on Cajal cells spread organs.

Part 05

Phlegm Mass Disorder Leads to Cirrhosis, Diabetes.

1

Septic Tank of our body! Middle Zone Disorder will lead to the pollution of whole body

Middle zone is like a dam door of a reservoir where water is kept to supply the field with water later. Once middle zone is polluted, whole body is susceptible to pollution. The dirty and murky blood kept in the middle zone is subjected to transfer to whole body immune system through blood vessels of outer walls of stomach and intestines, or lymphatic system, and blood vessel related diseases such as arteriosclerosis, metabolic diseases such as diabetes, toxic diseases such as skin trouble, and various infectious diseases. If the liver which is to detoxicate the stimulus is overburdened, toxic substance becomes even stronger and troubles our body.

The damaged mucous membrane eventually becomes the gate to let in toxic substances, and to cause lots of intractable diseases that has given no exact cause of outbreak, let alone to treat them such as autoimmune diseases, various metabolic syndrome, skin trouble such as atopy, sudden increase of type 2 diabetes, abdominal obesity, thyroid disease, joint diseases of unknown cause, and uterine disease. The circulation of toxin substance over the whole body brings each person different problems depending on the person's constitution and weak part.

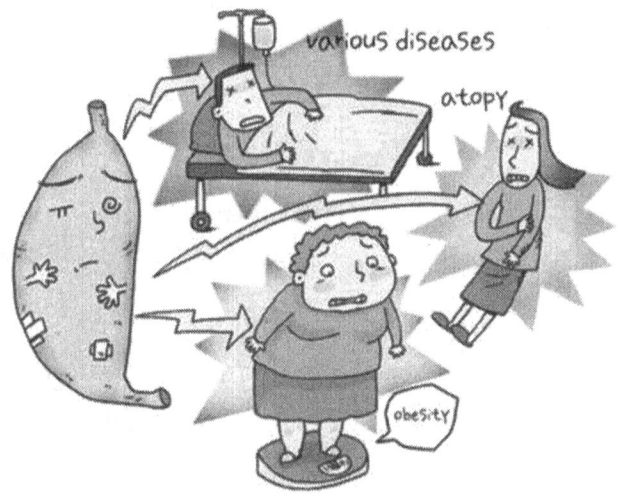

# 2

Change of whole body caused by phlegm mass disorder

The following data is the result of observations for 3 years and 12,000 clinical cases of phlegm mass disorder patients. It was to examine and record general symptoms they commonly complained. When phlegm mass disorder treatment was applied to these patients, they saw clinical results that most of the symptoms disappear or relieved. Therefore it is confirmed that causes of diseases in the below is phlegm mass disorder.

Disorder in water metabolism
body swelling up
significant abdominal obesity
diarrhea and constipation taking place irregularly
often catching nephrotic syndrome

Digestive system deteriorating
always feeling full and bloated though eating small
often having upset stomach and reflux
feeling heartburn or stomach cramps
having carsick, dry heaves, and vomit

often full of gas, poor bowel movements

often diagnosed neurogenic gastritis or irritable colon syndrome

Having disorder in reproductive organs

having severe menstrual pain

having irregular menstrual cycle, sometimes menopause

often having endometriosis, uterine myoma, vagina discharge, hysteritis

having bladder hardened, frequent urination, not feeling completed urination

often having cystitis with no reason

prostatic hypertrophy and prostate's syndrome

Unstable immune system, skin troubles

easily catching cold and infectious diseases

often having allergy on skin, nose, and bronchial tube

having chronic athletic foot and eczema

often catching autoimmune diseases such as Behcet's disease, arthritis

often having bruises in body, canker sore in mouth and tongue

having murky eyes, dark countenance, freckles

often having acne or breakouts

having dark circle

once skin cut, getting easily infected, getting boil easily

Waste caused murky blood influencing brain

having headache, dizziness

absentmindedness becoming worse, leading to dementia

having arteriosclerosis often

likely having high blood pressure and stroke

having dry eyes (xerophthalmia) or ophthalmalgia

having severe bad breath

Often having metabolism disorders

easily catching type 2 diabetes or hypoglycemia

always feeling fatigue and lethargy because of chronic fatigue syndrome

having hyperlipidemia and cirrhosis

having easy hepatitis virus multiplication, easy progress of hepatitis patient to cirrhosis

Having disorders in joint and muscles

having degenerative joint disease or making noise in joint when moving

having stiff nape neck and painful, intramuscular pain on shoulders and whole body

having back pain or cramp in the leg with no reason

having gout or nonspecific arthritis

Easy breaking up the balance between mind and body

becoming anxious and worried, getting angry over trifle things and annoyed

catching thyroid disease easily

catching depression easily

always feeling sleepy

feeling pressure on the chest, angina, short of breath like asthma

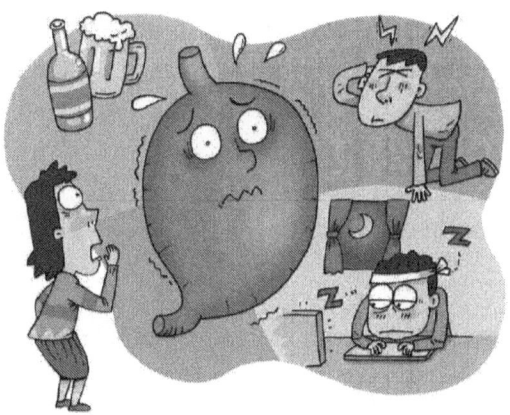

3

Major retractable diseases caused by phlegm mass disorder

As such, physiological function and organs of the whole body, influenced by the toxin of the phlegm mass disorder, undergo many symptoms and changes. If these pathological phenomena continue, they settle down as diseases. Following is the record of major diseases phlegm mass disorder patients experienced, but later their symptoms got improved through the phlegm mass disorder treatment, therefore proved the cause-and-effect relationship with the disorder. In addition, it presents the pathological mechanism how these diseases take place in what process and the concept of treatment is suggested.

Phlegm mass toxin that causes headache

'I have pounding headache,' 'I have splitting headache.' 'I have throbbing headache,' 'I have migraine.'

The kinds and extents of headaches patients feel are all different, but no medicine to cure headache has been developed yet. It is just to get over with painkillers. About 40% of world population complains severe headache. It is very common disease that no one is free from headache while living on earth. Why has no medicine been developed despite the cutting edge medical advancement of today? To put it simply, it is because fundamental cause of the headache has not been found. In this sense, finding of phlegm mass disorder has opened up a decisive way of searching for causative agent that causes headache.

The idea that phlegm mass toxin causes headache started when I had observed that phlegm mass disorder patients commonly complain headache. From old, oriental medicine explains that headache takes place because of stomach problems but it does not offer objective mechanism how it actually causes headache.

But the fact that degeneration of polluted middle zone cause phlegm mass disorder became proved right. Because of that, the mechanism of gastrointestinal tract causes headache and dizziness to take place. All the headaches, of course, are to blame on gastrointestinal tract problems. Stress or various elements may contribute to it, but the most part of the problems has something to do with phlegm mass toxin.

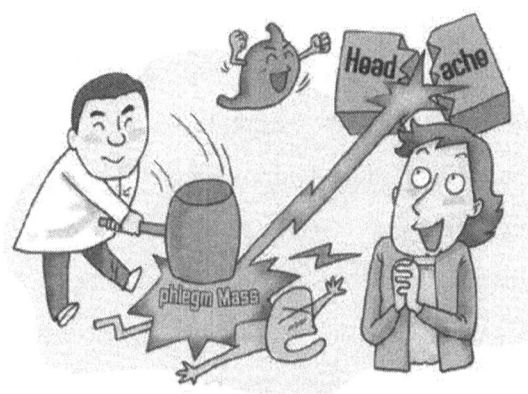

Most female patients who practically live on headache medicines have chronic indigestion problems. Though they complain that headache become worse when they have indigestion issue, they do not think of treating gastrointestinal tract, but habitually prefer to take headache medicines.

The reason of having headache when indigestion is because phlegm mass toxins, out of middle zone damage, influence nervous system or by direct infiltrating the brain through blood vessels that cause headache.

There are those who have no headache in case of indigestion, but there are also those who feel acute headache and dizziness in case they feel slight indigestion. It is connected to the extent of damage of mucous membrane. Those whose meshed tissue of gastrointestinal tract mucous membrane is severely destroyed, various toxins inside the stomach and intestines easily permeate and toxins swiftly spread over the whole body, headache or dizziness appear whenever indigestion becomes the issue.

Controlling phlegm mass so does dizziness

People generally think that dizziness comes because of anemia, but most of it has to do with toxin in brain and ears. Brain toxin caused dizziness is in line with headache. Especially the ear problem caused dizziness is connected to phlegm mass disorder.

Meniere disease that shows spasmodical dizziness, otolith, the tiny little stone that rolls inside the ears and cause dizziness but has no cure except to make patients get used to the symptoms, and lymphedema, the ear related dizziness are all caused by influences from phlegm mass toxins formed in gastrointestinal tract.

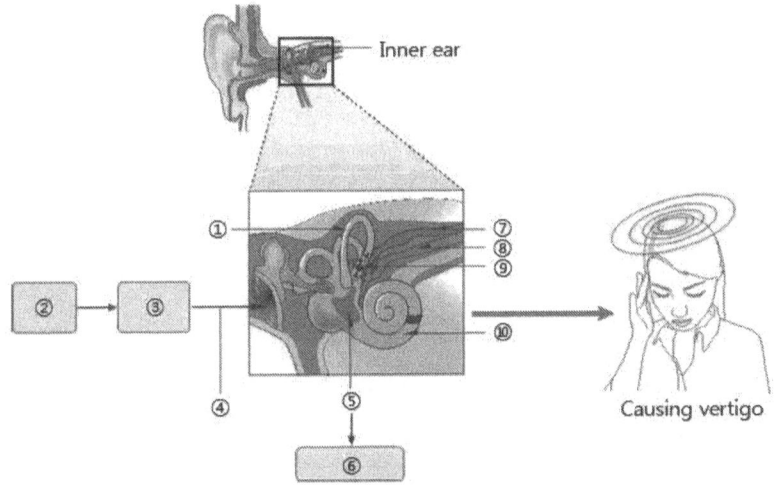

①Semicircular ducts ②Phlegm accumulation syndrome ③Phlegm toxic ④Circulatory disturbance of endolymph and bacterial multiplication ⑤Endolymphatic hydrops ⑥Meniere's disease ⑦Vestibular nerve ⑧Cochlear nerve ⑨Development of otolith ⑩Cochlear canal

Ears are exposed to water smearing inside when taking shower or shampooing. But the water inside does not have to be intentionally drained out. It is drained with the self-cleaning capacity. Problems arise when the self-cleaning capacity gets broken. When phlegm mass toxin once delivered to ears from gastrointestinal tract, the inner ears become damp and moisture cleaning capacity lowered, and therefore various germs grow and inflammation develops. The polluted moisture kept in the bottom and form lymphedema, if continues, it is made to toxic node to cause dizziness. Therefore, ear caused dizziness is also related to gastrointestinal tract. That is why ear related dizziness is treated with medicines of promoting water metabolism, in oriental medicine.

Phlegm mass disorder treatment aims at fundamental treatment of diabetes.

8% of whole population is diabetes patients. 300 thousands new patients are added each year. Among the OECD member countries, diabetes related death rate is number one. This is the current picture of diabetes in Korea. Diabetes is a disease either pancreas does not secrete insulin properly or glucose is not used appropriately and it is stored in blood vessels. Its complication is more dangerous than disease itself. If glucose is not managed properly and high glucose status continues for long, it harms each organ of the body as it travels along the blood vessels and cause to lose eyesight (diabetic retinopathy), to amputate leg (leg ulcers), to cause renal failure, stroke, and peripheral circulatory disturbance.

Compared to its severity, the medical response to it is inadequate. Most of diabetes treatment nowadays aims to manage the disease, not to bring complete treatment. But continuous taking of medication may cause insulin resistance and weakening of pancreas cells. Type 2 diabetes is not insulin related. It has enough insulin, but does not consume glucose and therefore glucose sets in blood vessels. The reason is those tissue cell membranes get polluted by wastes. This triggers the insulin censor capacity lowered and resistance to insulin, and eventually makes the glucose inflow to tissue cell drops.

The waste that sets in tissue cell membrane is called 'dahm' (phlegm) in oriental medicine. This 'dahm' is made and delivered from phlegm mass disorder.

The phlegm mass toxin seems to damage pancreas also. When phlegm mass toxin gets accumulated in pancreas, antigen substance is produced in pancreas and this causes autoimmune phenomenon that destroy pancreas cells and leads to insulin production disorder.

It has been proved that phlegm mass toxin is the main cause of type 2 diabetes by the following clinical case. In order to remove the waste in cell membrane, phlegm mass removal method was applied which is detox purification therapy practiced by oriental medicine and alternative medicine. When phlegm mass gets removed from gastrointestinal tract outer walls, blood sugar drops even when hypoglycemic agent or insulin intake lowered or stopped, it shows treatment effect.

A 43 year old female pyknic type patient whose cholesterol level was 1,250 and more than 200 on fasting blood sugar, when hospitalized, after phlegm mass treatment, her fasting blood sugar dropped below 100, and therefore stopped taking the diabetes medication and cholesterol level also dropped below 300. Her general health condition observed to be enhanced. Such clinical case proves that wrong eating habit and obesity caused 'acquired diabetes' has something to do with phlegm mass disorder.

Blood sugar control principles by way of phlegm mass treatment
* removing wastes contained in tissue cell membrane
* promoting insulin production of pancreas cells
* activating enhanced glucose metabolism process of liver
* in severe diabetes case, using hypoglycemic agent and insulin medication of western medicine combined, gradually control the medication

Cirrhosis, the hardening of liver, is it because of phlegm mass toxin?

Liver disease constitutes #1 cause of death of Korean males in their forties. Cirrhosis, the typical life threatening disease for Korean males in their forties and fifties, when becoming serious, complications take place and proceed to liver cancer. It is reported that the major cause of cirrhosis is as following: B type hepatitis 68%, C type hepatitis 15%, and alcoholic hepatitis 17%. Fortunately, with the help of preventative vaccination, outbreak of B type hepatitis is decreased, but hepatitis patients proceeding to cirrhosis has been sharply increased. This puts seriousness on the issue. Outbreak of hepatitis is decreasing, but why does the case of hepatitis developing to cirrhosis increasing up to 30 to 60%?

Oriental medicine sees the reason of hardening of liver as the patients' wrong eating habits, anger, fatigue, repeated over-drinking, especially when leading a life of gluttonous, overeating, sporadic overeating, and eating at late night leads to undigested nutrition get accumulated in the body, and it will be toxins to influence the liver and later cause the outbreak of cirrhosis. The cirrhosis is not only influenced by hepatitis virus, but also by blood toxins and pollution that is coming from gastrointestinal tract. Therefore the cirrhosis is also directly connected to gastrointestinal tract outer walls, in other words, the conditions of middle zone. The middle zone functions as cleaning agent of blood to send to liver. Its problems are directly delivered to liver. In actuality, liver cells can be hardened anytime even though it does not show in blood test or supersonic test. Phlegm mass can function as a cause to deteriorate hepatitis diseases. A simple hepatitis carrier who did not worry about the case all of a sudden find out that his case developed to cirrhosis, because of this mechanism.

It is no exaggeration, therefore, to say that pollution in the middle zone is the core element in the development to the cirrhosis. In the late 2005, a patient of late stage cirrhosis and liver cancer came to me. I applied the phlegm mass disorder treatment to the patient for the first time. The patient was diagnosed by a hospital doctors and told to be able to live up to only 2 or 3 months. The patient lives a relatively healthy life even after 2 years have passed since then. I applied this phlegm mass disorder treatment to all patients with malignant liver diseases. As expected, I could witness the livers becoming greatly activated because of middle zone purification treatment in which the entering blood got cleansed. When examining the patients with cirrhosis or liver cancer, I could see how their phlegm mass disorder was far worse than any other patients. It stresses out the importance of what and how to eat.

When phlegm mass is removed and cleansed blood sent to there, the liver, though it cannot say a word, would dance, I explain. The liver used to receive dirty and polluted blood, but now cleansed blood it receives. How much can the liver cells feel pleasant? As is well known, liver has the strongest regenerating capacity. Even with the slightest help, it will make the most of the rest of capacity and restore the full capacity by itself.

Arteriosclerosis also starts from phlegm mass

Stroke is the result of cerebrovascular gets blocked or exploded. We may think that the stroke has nothing to do with gastrointestinal tract. But think about these! Low blood pressure patient with weak gastrointestinal tract at one point gradually increase the blood pressure and the stroke breakout. Or someone with too strong stomach who always claimed he had no problem no matter how much he ate, started having arteriosclerosis and high blood pressure and at one point got stroke. How can we explain these?

Further study should be done to clarify this, but I believe that phlegm mass toxin gets accumulated in the blood vessels and the vessels get hardened. As we have seen so far, wherever phlegm mass toxin gets accumulated, no matter it is muscle system or lymphatic system, it is degenerated in the form of hardening. (Shoulders become hardened because of the dahm, intramuscular pain, liver cells hardened to proceed to cirrhosis, and gastrointestinal tract outer walls hardened). Likewise, by phlegm mass toxin, whole body as well as blood vessels of brain can be also hardened and lose its resilience. This is the true nature of arteriosclerosis. When blood vessel loses its resilience and get hardened, the vessel cannot hold the rising blood pressure and receive damage. In this sense, stroke is related to phlegm mass toxin stored in gastrointestinal tract.

There was a 69 year old female patient in Summer 2004 who was diagnosed with brain hemorrhage, got operation, and hospitalized for 14 months, She was barely saved but did not get better, and later transferred to this hospital. She was unconscious by that time, and could not move her limbs. Oriental medicine stroke therapy was applied, but she showed no sign of moving her limbs. A month was wasted by the time I noticed that her phlegm mass toxin issue was severe. For the first time, I started applying the phlegm mass treatment to the stroke patient. The patient had suffered constipation for a long time, they said. As soon as the treatment started, she defecated all over the bed sheet. Later, she began moving her fingers and toes and started murmuring. A couple months of rehabilitation and the phlegm mass treatment made her recognize others around and she was able to raise her hands to her shoulder height. Because of her long suffering constipation, the phlegm mass toxins accumulated in the gastrointestinal tract outer walls spread and stored in blood vessel of brain, brain cells, muscles and blood vessel of limbs.

When problem happens in stomach and intestines, amnesia and dementia may follow

Why do we become forgetful (amnesia) as we get older? It is natural to become forgetful and memory power decrease. More important memory replaces less important ones. But most people fear that their forgetfulness may develop further into dementia. Until recently it was generally believed that forgetfulness and dementia are completely different issues and have no relations between the two. But recent studies show that the more forgetful one becomes, the more possibility of dementia one gets. People with severe forgetfulness become anxious about the issue.

How then do amnesia and dementia related? Surprisingly, both amnesia and dementia have relations with gastrointestinal tract. Over there, immune battle is always going on against various kinds of foods we take, and therefore pathological immune byproducts are also produced. This is called 'pathological immune cytokine.' The more we are exposed to overeating or polluted foods, the more pathological cytokine is produced. These cytokine damage the neurons and lower the brain capacity. Besides this, if phlegm mass toxin gets accumulated in the connective tissues with neurons, neurotransmission cannot be properly performed and therefore brain function gets lowered and amnesia happens. When the accumulation continues, the degeneration of neurons progresses and that leads to dementia.

In oriental medicine, 'phlegm and retained fluid,' the toxin produced in gastrointestinal tract, will attack brain area and it is regarded as the natural pathological phenomenon. Brain, in return, is to do physiological defense work, but if brain capacity has become weak because of fatigues, or too much toxin is to be made in gastrointestinal tract, the brain will gradually become polluted by the toxin. Then the amnesia and dementia can be called brain pollution caused by the gastrointestinal tract.

What if phlegm mass toxin reaches kidney?

Nephrotic syndrome is the complication of four symptoms; continuing of severe proteinuria, hypoalbuminemia, hyperlipidemia, and anasarca. Visible symptom is edema. In the early stage, it is as mild as eyelids swollen and can be ignored. When legs and top of the foot become swollen and can't put on shoes, or notice socks mark on the legs, and trousers become too small, one notices the kidney problems. The progress of symptoms all varies. Sometimes proteinuria naturally disappears, but the protein in the blood decrease, especially the albumin of the blood, and resistance to infection weakened, and may cause the breakout of pneumonia, urinary tract infection, and of blood poisoning that may lead to risk life. Fortunately, kidney is the only organ that comes with two pieces among all internal organs of our body. When one gets degenerated the other will make up the failure. But once damaged, unlike the liver, it is difficult to get restored. It is necessary to take care of kidney syndrome but also to strengthen the weakened kidney. Phlegm mass disorder treatment can make it strong.

For kidney, In order to perform the waste filtering work well, water metabolism should be done well. Kidney takes care of downstream of the water metabolism. Upstream is gastrointestinal tract. Most of the food we take is in the form of moisture. Taking food means to take water. The first part food comes into is the gastrointestinal tract. Therefore water metabolism takes place in the gastrointestinal tract in the first and in the biggest scale. If water metabolism does not take place properly and therefore polluted moisture goes down the tract, the kidney slowly gets polluted and damaged.

Arthritis – no known medical cause, blood with phlegm mass toxin flows through joints

Rheumatoid arthritis is what immune cells of our body mistakes the cells of our own body as foreign object and destroys them, the autoimmune disease. The prevalence of the disease is 1% of the population. It mostly attacks the joints of both limbs and cause chronic arthritis. If neglected, 70% patients will have deformed joints in hands and feet. After 20 years, more than 60% will be limited to basic self-administration of them or need assistance in all of their activities. It is reported that 7 out of 10 rheumatoid arthritis patients stopped their job because they did not receive treatment on time.

If the disease stays long, complication incidence rises such as various infectious diseases, cardiovascular diseases, and lymphoma. Average life expectancy is reduced by 7 to 10 years. As is most of autoimmune diseases, rheumatoid arthritis also has no known causes. There is no way of complete treatment or prevention of the disease. Especially, cause of the following diseases are almost unknown; rheumatoid similar diseases such as spondylarthritis ankylopoietica, systemic lupus erythematosus, or gout, tendonitis, aponeurositis, and bursitis,

Oriental medicine recognizes most of arthritis as internal medicine disease. When the blood circulating to joints becomes murky, the high viscosity blood gets accumulated in joints and causes germs and viruses increase or it damages the joint fluids. Therefore treatment is focused on moist heat, cold-damp, removal of extravasated blood, and promoting blood circulation. In the oriental medicine, the reason blood gets polluted and murky are various. But the main reason is the phlegm mass toxin that is formed in gastrointestinal tract. The toxic material of the middle zone is sent to the whole body through the blood vessel and lymphoid organ on the gastrointestinal tract. It is the same dirty and murky blood that reaches the joints, and damages various autoimmune response and the joints. When phlegm mass toxin removal treatment was applied to a multiple joint arthritis patient, the swelling red and inflammatory symptom stopped worsening. Therefore removing of phlegm mass toxin, taking unpolluted food, and applying professional joint treatments, intractable joint diseases are expected to improve.

Death causing depression

WHO predicted that depression would be the number 2 disease to torment the humanity by the year 2020. About 3.2 million people suffer from depression in Korea every year. One person at every 45 minutes loses life by committing suicide. 80% of them had suffered depression. When serious, it may cause killing oneself. Most people take it as slight mood change and can be overcome with determination. But depression is clearly a disease. It is also caused by physical problem.

A patient who once tried to commit suicide says that he found himself to stand on the edge of a river, glancing at the water surface, he was compelled to jump into the water. The fact that he tried to commit suicide away from his will shows that depression is not the matter of emotion only but it is rooted either on nervous system or hormone system. It means that it is physical problem.

Middle zone of gastrointestinal tract is called the second brain. It has more nervous cells than the spinal cord, the nervous organ. Countless number of neurotransmitter which was believed to be made only in brain is secreted there. The hormone 'serotonin' prevents depression and 90% of serotonin is secreted in gastrointestinal tract. The greatest obstruction to secretion of serotonin is the change of gastrointestinal tract environment by the toxin and damage the nervous system of the stomach and intestines. In the clinical case, when removal of toxin treatment applied, patients felt that their body lightened and depression relieved. This proves that gastrointestinal tract toxin directly related to the outbreak of depression. These facts are by all means new and important. Depression is not only about mental or nervous system issue, but also about wrong eating habit or about gastrointestinal tract being polluted by inflow of toxins. This understanding of depression is expected to open a new horizon in treating depression.

Alcohol addicts and phlegm mass disorder

Alcohol issue has been a big issue traditionally, but its seriousness is beyond the acceptable level. Excess drinking causes early death and declining of productivity, and therefore its socioeconomic cost is about 17 billion dollars. It is equivalent to making a new city or to the defense budget for a year. As Victor Hugo said, God made water, manmade wine. Alcohol has been with humanity in history. But the issue is about alcohol addiction. Moderate drinking makes the relationship smooth and pleasant. If it is too much, however, it is not man drinks alcohol, but the other way around.

Normal food is digested and fermented and transferred to suitable format to become absorbed in the cells of our body. In the meantime, we may feel full and satisfied and therefore cannot eat much. But alcohol is taken as it is already fermented and absorbed fast into cells. However, stomach and intestines do not feel full and satisfied and therefore keep drinking even though we get drunk, it is easy to get addicted to alcohol this way.

From medical point of view, this is how one gets addicted to alcohol. Early stage of alcoholic addict starts from excess accumulation of fat on liver. In the middle stage, oxygen consumption increase as liver cells deal with excess alcohol. It then makes liver cells suffer from lack of oxygen. Liver cells destroyed fast from this stage.

Between liver cells and portal vein, the nutrition supply channel, there is well developed thin connective tissues that sustain the liver. Excess alcohols and 'not-detoxicated' phlegm mass toxins that are kept in portal vein flow to these connective tissues. Those inflow alcohol elements and phlegm mass toxins make the connective tissues hardened and increase. The whole liver becomes degenerated to fibrosis. This is cirrhosis. When person with severe phlegm mass toxin drinks lots of alcohol, the liver cells get easily hardened and proceed to cirrhosis.

Those degenerated to 'fibrosis' connective cells and surrounding nervous tissues, because it is degenerated by alcohol and toxins, continue to ask for more alcohol and even send false information to brain in order to receive alcohol. It develops to abnormal mental response.

If central nervous system is controlled by alcohol, it is now alcohol that behaves as master of the body. Once alcohol becomes the master of the body and the body is controlled by alcohol, it is called 'alcohol addicted.'

Medical treatment of alcoholic addiction has been on mental counselling, IV with vitamin supply, and tranquillizer at the most. It has low rate of treatment and cannot be a fundamental treatment.

The genuine treatment of alcohol addict should be, as in the above, from removing the alcohol and phlegm mass toxins that have been formed in liver connective tissues and nervous system. Once the accumulated alcohol toxins and phlegm mass toxins are removed, those alcohol depending nerve cells become normal and asking alcohol less, fibrosis connective tissues resolved, and if not severe last stage, liver can be restored to normality to some degree.

In clinical practice, to severe case alcohol addicted cirrhosis patients, I applied phlegm mass toxin removal treatment and administered 'hepacure,' most of the patients said that they did not desire for the alcohol anymore and showed normal range in liver function test. Some patients even returned to their job.

Serious food addiction! Stress caused heavy eating

Addiction is not limited to alcohols only. Food addiction is almost the same as alcohol addiction. Some do not eat when stressed, but others eat recklessly. The latter lost the ability of restrain the appetite because of the stress. If this becomes a habit, one eats heavy even when stress is not the issue. Alcohol addicted patient may recognize the seriousness of the issue and tries to stop drinking, but one is already inclined to drink it anyway. The one who used to overeating, naturally look for food regardless of one's willingness. Those food addicted patients may suffer from chronic indigestion and obesity and develop to adult diseases such as arteriosclerosis and diabetes.

Overeating and sporadic heavy eating that need to be corrected for the sake of health can also be solved by phlegm mass disorder treatment. Overeating and sporadic heavy eating proceed to phlegm mass disorder in the following manner. Holding on to the bad eating habit makes the meshed up tissues of gastrointestinal tract mucous membrane damaged chronically and brings middle zone damage in return. If overeaten food wastes flow into the middle zone, splanchnic nervous system gets degenerated and asks for more food. This false information influences the central nervous system of the brain and proceeds to food addiction that can't wait for the food. Stress caused heavy eaters and those who keep eating habitually are suffering from same addiction as alcohol addicts, though the substance of the addiction is different. It is the result of addiction to food by being degenerated of splanchnic nervous system and central nervous system.

The cause of autism can be also phlegm mass toxin

In the States, the number of autistic children gradually increases, and it becomes one out of 150 children. As in the Korean movie 'Marathon,' the patient is trapped in one's own world, and can't communicate with others. Living a normal social life is difficult. Since the person needs someone's help always, all family members feel it difficult. It is not known yet how autism takes place. It is only known that it happens when sense relation part of cerebral nerves gets damaged. I want to suggest that autism also has connection to gastrointestinal tract.

Damage on mucous epithelial cells of gastrointestinal tract or immune disorder creates intestinal bacteria. The bacteria in return create exorphine which is comprised of gliadorphine and casomorphine. These elements are not absorbed, but excreted. If these are absorbed to inside the body through intestines, they enter central nervous system and engage in creating endorphin which makes people feeling good. This is yet a hypothesis, but it can suggest the possibility of intestinal damage may end in brain damage. In clinical case, half of autistic children complain of intestinal disorder such as defecating watery stool or having often diarrhea, Out of this, we cannot definitely say that intestinal disorder cause autism, but it shows some correlation. Some substances from neurological damage in the intestines are absorbed in the body and set in brain can cause mental disorder. Precise mechanism is to be studied further but it is certain that the condition of gastrointestinal tract has relations with clinical condition of autism. It is expected that before autism related brain neurological section get damaged, we may prevent the progress of autism to some extent by controlling some elements of gastrointestinal tract.

Phlegm mass toxin, enemy of Behcet's disease, the rare intractable disease

Behcet's disease is a whole body multiple chronic inflammatory disease. It has symptoms of recurrent skin ulcer, canker sore, pudenda ulcer, digestive system ulcer, keratitis, conjunctivitis, uveitis, and whole body arthritis. It may result in losing eyesight or brain damage, the rare intractable disease. In Korea, the first Behcet's disease was reported in 1961. Its patients continue to increase since 1980. On why the disease outbreaks, some hypothesis are suggested as following: caused by virus, or by pesticide or heavy metals, by gene related, or by immune disorder. Among all those, immune related one is the most convincing, the autoimmune theory, the medical circle sees.

Autoimmune disease is an immune response that refuses the substance that has been created in the body and in the process from inflammation or ulcer. Antigen is created in the body that attacks its own body. The reason of this phenomenon is believed that environment of body is polluted by various causes and lots of harmful materials are formed. These harmful substances function as antigen. Our body is polluted because of sharply increasing polluted food, environment and water pollution, heavy metals, pesticides, harmful food additives, preservatives, bleaches, and various drug poisons. The most ideal treatment of Behcet's disease, therefore, is to improve the environment of body so that antigen, the enemy of autoimmune response, is not to be made. Improving of poisonous body environment starts, of course, from removing of phlegm mass toxins. When purifying the poisonous environment by removing the phlegm mass toxins, the body does not make antigen material and therefore autoimmune response is not to be proceeded.

Removing of phlegm mass toxin does not solve Behcet's disease. Oriental medicine thinks that the strongest cause of

Behcet's disease is 'liver fever' or 'liver moist heat.' Stress, fatigue, alcohol, and chemical liver toxin create the liver environment and lead the whole body immune response in its excess. The excess immune takes slightest harmful element to engage immune war, not the 'immune tolerance,' and inflict inflammations, ulcers, and tissue damages in the whole body. In a word, Behcet's disease is thought to be created in the basis of phlegm mass toxin and by the liver fever.

In the clinical case, for a 45 years male Behcet's disease patient who suffered from canker sore, genital ulcer, and multiple arthritis, I administered phlegm mass disorder treatment and liver fever restraint therapy. As a result, canker sore disappeared, eye pain and genital ulcer diminished, and the severe arthritis that needed to take 6 pills a day significantly improved as much as to stop taking the pills.

Various treatments have been tried to cure Behcet's disease, but no satisfactory medication has been developed yet. The pills used so far were mostly strong medications such as immunosuppressant. It may treat symptoms but leave side effects that it is hard to use long term. Further study needs to be done, but phlegm mass disorder treatment that aims to improve the poisonous environment, and liver fever restraint therapy that controls excess immune response, are expected to become a new treatment model for Behcet's disease in the future.

Atopy - polluted skin by phlegm mass toxin

'Depressed about atopy and killed oneself.' 'Resolved to immigrate for the sake of atopy suffering child'

People may not believe those news pieces about killing oneself because of atopy and immigrate to abroad. But its distress level is beyond one's imagination. Etymology of atopy is 'strange,' 'mysterious.' and 'unfamiliar.' As is implied in the etymology, it is hard to cure the disease. Therefore, patients may try one clinic to another and depend on unproven therapies and make the case worse. As for how atopy outbreak, it is believed that dust, polluted environment, instant food, and various modern day issues trigger the disease, but no reason is pinpointed. I believe that along with proper medication, if phlegm mass disorder treatment is administered, it will be overcome! Through skin, sweats and other wastes are discharged. The skin functions as an excretory organ, and therefore wastes of the body are continually flowing to skin. If it cannot deal with the wastes properly, skin degeneration begins. The more phlegm mass toxin, the worse skin degeneration becomes. Phlegm mass toxin impedes the blood circulation in the skin. Mucus helps skin soft, but phlegm mass toxin makes it diminish or polluted. Phlegm mass toxin makes the immune function too sensitive. It causes severe irritation, bacteria increase in the skin, dry skin, and darkened or undergo cornification. Therefore the severe chronic skin diseases are caused by phlegm mass toxin or polluted substances. It is far important to deal with the origin of the skin pollution.

A 41 years old male patient came to this clinic with unbearable itching, dark and rough skin. He was said to be overburdened with his work. He was used to eat fast food and instant food, and got used to sporadic overeating and eating fast. Atopy skin appeared 10 years ago. His phlegm mass disorder was serious. I started removing phlegm mass toxin which had been spread all over his body along with fasting treatment. With several months of treatment, his face became cleansed, and his festered back and hands became clean. He was able to maintain almost normal skin. At the moment, he renovates his eating habits, and says that he experiences lightened body and skin.

Besides these, phlegm mass toxin spread all over our body and cause lots symptoms and diseases; bad breath, shoulders pain, intramuscular pain, uterine myoma, chronic uterus inflammation, frequent cystitis, prostate hypertrophy, thyroid nodule, and hypothyroidism are linked to phlegm mass disorder. Clear mechanism is not yet available, but the following diseases look triggered by phlegm mass toxin; gastrointestinal tract related cancers such as gastric cancer, colon cancer, esophageal cancer, and uterine cancer, breast cancer, thyroid cancer, and pancreatic cancer.

As we have seen, lots of diseases we have known are caused by bad way of eating, the one we unconsciously perform every day. Many diseases are made on dining table. It may look too simple that we may ignore the importance. With the discovery of middle zone and phlegm mass disorder, however, it has become major cause of disease. Especially the dining speed of Koreans is 3 times faster than that of people of other countries. Korea is vulnerable country to phlegm mass disorder, and we should not neglect on eating habit most of all. If Koreans keep the principle of 'slow and chew well', the troublesome and intractable diseases that put many of them under chronic, malign, and intractable disease will be far less than now.

Part 06

Diagnosis and Treatment of Phlegm Mass Disorder: Self-Diagnosis of it

Phlegm mass disorder self-diagnosis check list

* gas filled inside and bloating
* defecating but feeling incomplete
* often feeling headache
* having dizziness
* having dim eyesight
* feeling dry and painful around eyes
* becoming more absent minded
* looking pale, dark and having freckles
* having stiff nape of neck
* having intramuscular pain on shoulders
* always feeling fatigued
* having bad breath
* for women, often having peripheral vascular circulation disorder & inflammation
* often having upset stomach
* feeling nauseous at the stomach
* often reflux

One item gets one point

More than 10 points: very serious status

5 to 9 points: serious status

Below 4: not serious status

Tests to diagnose phlegm mass disorder

Abdomen exam to evaluate the hardness of gastrointestinal tract outer walls in 12 stages	**X-ray on abdomen** to examine the condition and location of stool and gas
Blood test (when necessary) when to examine the liver function and check other diseases	**Meridian function test** to examine the function of stomach and intestines and to check the extent of toxins
Phlegm mass disorder survey designed to clarify the nature of phlegm mass disorder of the patient	**Phlegm mass toxin tester** to evaluate the hardness of gastrointestinal tract outer walls with ultrasonic waves

1

Treatment of phlegm mass disorder

By discovering the middle zone and phlegm mass disorder, new way of curing unknown disease, a gastrointestinal tract disorder, is open! Besides, the phlegm mass disorder was thought to be just a gastrointestinal outer wall problem but it has become known that it is the cause of so many whole body diseases. Naturally, the way of treating the lesion on the gastrointestinal tract has to be changed. Now it is not about removing inflammation and covering ulcers anymore. It is more about scrutinizing and improving all the organs that constitute the gastrointestinal tract. This attitude is to go beyond the superficial problems such as inflammations or ulcers and improve the background and environment of gastrointestinal tract that cause real problems. This is more fundamental solution.

The core of background treatment is from natural logic that says the environment inside the gastrointestinal tract is similar with earth and swamp of the nature.

For example, oriental medicine name a disease called 'stomach moist heat.' When caused by overeating and over drinking, the disease appears in the form of indigestion, nausea, headache, dizziness, and urination becomes darker and body feels heavy. Moist heat is damp and humid atmosphere, in other words, it is like in the rainy season when ventilation is bad, and mold and bacteria easily increase. This kind of natural moist heat environment can be created by overeating and drinking alcohol. Once moist heat environment created, bacteria increased in the gastrointestinal tract, immune system degenerated, and various pathological cytokine to appear to make inflammation, ulcer, and various functional gastrointestinal tract symptoms. Upon this logic, middle zone damage repairing treatment is administered. This is the basis of phlegm mass disorder treatment.

Grafting the middle zone study of western medicine into the pathological concept of gastrointestinal tract of oriental medicine has made a new way of treatment, a very important medical victory.

Now we need to shift the treatment focus from mucus damage repair to apprehend the degenerated environment or pathological condition accurately and to improve this condition. For example, we need to approach the treatment differently by improving inside the polluted gastrointestinal tract, softening the hardened muscles, removing toxins stuck in immune system and nervous system, and making the blocked or narrowed blood trafficking smooth, quite different way from gastrointestinal tract treatment in the past.

In the beginning of developing treatment, in order to remove phlegm mass, we administered various ways and naturopathy such as, digestive enzymes, medicine for promoting digestion, medicine for removing phlegm mass, fasting, and bowel cleansing. Most of them did not accomplish the purpose. Symptoms got better but the hardened tissues were not softened. Once treatment stopped, the disease reoccurred. Through the trials and errors, we have come up with the understanding that the nature of phlegm mass disorder is more complicated pathological changes than the abdominal mass or retention of indigested food oriental medicine speaks. Therefore we stopped the treatment practice with removing food stagnation that tried to break up the hardened tissue masses. Instead, we clarified all the possible problem patterns that may happen on the gastrointestinal tract outer wall and interpreted each case in oriental medicine terms and considered all the cases to develop the phlegm mass disorder treatment and finally softened the hardening phenomena of outer wall.

1. Principles of phlegm mass disorder treatment

1) Improving the environment of gastrointestinal tract polluted with bacteria, germs and food wastes
2) Normalizing immune response by improving pathological cytokine
3) Promoting restoration of pathological environment by boosting blood circulation
4) Activating movements of gastrointestinal tract by loosening up the smooth muscle
5) Strengthening mucous membrane function by providing mucus and softening the hardened tissues
6) Loosening up the phlegm mass of stomach and large intestine with hot medicine in nature, because they are cold mass,

small intestine with cold medicine, because it is hot in nature

7) Administering western medicine prescription in case of mucous membrane disease of severe ulcer and inflammation,

2. Phlegm mass disorder treatment

The phlegm mass disorder treatment that treats the gastrointestinal tract outer wall is obviously a new medical challenge. As we have experienced lots of trials and errors on our way of developing, it is not a simple treatment. But by grafting the western and oriental medicine to consider the degenerated status of middle zone and develop the phlegm mass disorder curing medicine, the new way of treating the disease began opening. For the advanced case patients and for those who have complications with mental disorder because of the phlegm mass, in order to maximize the removing the phlegm mass toxins, we have supplemented the technics of alternative medicine and have structured the following comprehensive program.

1) Herbal medicine

This research team has developed 'phlegm mass solution 1,2,3.' They are for the people of weakness type, of heat in the excess type, and of vital energy deficiency type. These medicines are designed according to each patient's physical constitution and nature of phlegm mass. These will be the very first medications that are designed to treat gastrointestinal tract outer wall treatments, we believe. For the people of weakness type, it is used for cold physical constitution or for the phlegm mass mostly in the stomach and large intestines. For the people of heat in the excess type, it is for those whose phlegm mass mostly in small intestine or there is hot natured constipation in large intestine. And for the people of vital energy deficiency type, it is for those whose heart is too weak to supply the gastrointestinal tract with proper amount of blood, and therefore lack mucus on the gastrointestinal tract and the phlegm mass become as hard as stone.

2) Western medicine

Phlegm mass solutions are for improving the gastrointestinal tract outer wall. If mucous membrane damage is severe, applying the solutions may cause reverse effect. Mucous membrane, of inside, damage is better to be treated with western medicine. By taking care of mucous membrane by western medicine and outer wall by herbal medicine, we treat both inside and out and can be a fundamental remedy for gastrointestinal tract treatment.

3) Herbal acupuncture therapy

It is to graft meridian system theory of oriental medicine and herbal medicine theory and to put herbal medicine extract through meridian points to cure the disease. Herbal acupuncture therapy for phlegm mass is to put the herbal extract directly to the outer wall of gastrointestinal tract through the meridian points of the abdomen. It is to enhance the effect of therapy and shorten the treatment period.

4) Moxibustion therapy, bean curd pack therapy, & coffee enema therapy

* Moxibustion therapy – It is to put moxibustion on the phlegm mass area of gastrointestinal tract outer wall to induce the blood circulation and provide yang (plus) energy to dissolve ice like phlegm mass, and to activate the intestinal toxins.

* Bean curd pack therapy – It is to activate the intestinal movements to remove the feces from the intestines when administering fasting therapy to severe phlegm mass disorder patients, bean curd pack therapy will relax the hardened intestines and ease the breathing and urinating.

* Coffee enema therapy – Dr. Max Gerson invented the therapy and has been used for more than 70 years as ways of treatment of diseases and dieting. Its safety is proven. The program uses organic coffee. It helps to remove the long remaining feces from intestines, to improve the liver function, and to remove toxins by absorbing potassium from intestines and sending it to liver through blood vessels.

Besides this, following therapies have been developed; Liver purification therapy is to activate the detoxication capacity of liver. Leg bath therapy is to stimulate the feet, 'the second heart,' with hot water. It helps the blood circulation of the whole body and energizes the circulation of the Qi (energy) and normalizes the functions of autonomic nerves. Aroma mixed cold and hot water interchanging bath (it is to purify lymph to strengthen the immune response, to repeat the contraction and relaxation of vascular muscle to promote the blood circulation, and to stimulate the skin). Helium neon laser acupuncture therapy that provides the blood with low laser energy (it is to make the biological responses in the blood, such as enzyme response and oxidation reduction response, to happen smoothly to strengthen immune capacity and help various treatments of diseases). Resonance therapy (Normalizing metabolism and immune system of the body and removing the fundamental cause of diseases to restore back to heath by using GI – 2000, IR emitter) Eating raw therapy (Foods are manufactured from grain, vegetable, and seaweeds being treated at minimum level, not cooked at high temperature, but prepared in freeze drying or low temperature drying to avoid meat diet, instant food, and processed food that have caused various chronic diseases.)

TIP: Is my gastrointestinal tract a highway to bathroom?

Going to bathroom as soon as eating something is a protection mechanism of our body. It may be a nervous system mechanism to excrete excess food to outside of body or when having experienced severe stomach upset, nerves remember the food and sensitively react when it comes in again. In oriental medicine, it happens when there is retention of undigested food, before it becomes phlegm-retention syndrome or phlegm mass disorder after taking excess food or having aftereffect of upset stomach. The symptom may disappear when treating the retention of undigested food or having liquid food for some time.

2

Our body this much changed when phlegm mass disorder treated

As we have seen, phlegm mass disorder is the source of so many diseases. We humans are to live by eating all the time. Therefore what and how we eat is of crucial importance; wrong way of eating and eating polluted food cause the blood of our body murky, this blood gradually damages the blood, immune, nerves, and muscle systems and all organs and develop all kinds of diseases.

With the discovery of phlegm mass disorder, we have understood the background of the toxins and how it flows to influence other organs. Therefore, diagnosis and treatment of phlegm mass disorder has offered basis of treating lots of diseases. The following is the clinical record of benefits from treating the phlegm mass disorder.

Stomach and colon cancer, the nation's most frequent cancer, can be much reduced!

Why is it that Koreans have more stomach cancer than other kinds? Some say that salty and spicy food is to be blamed. Recent research says, however, that capsaicin, the main ingredient of hot pepper, is rather helpful to prevent the stomach cancer. It is not right to put spicy food responsible for the kind of cancer.

Examining the pathological status of phlegm mass disorder, the dirty environment phlegm mass creates is more likely causing the problem, and therefore the main cause of creating the phlegm mass, eating fast, overeating, sporadic overeating, and polluted food, is the background of stomach cancer. With these reasons, by treating phlegm mass disorder or eating food slowly and chew well, just by changing the way of eating, can we reduce the stomach cancer incidence significantly.

Opening a new era in preventing and treatment of dementia!

Alzheimer's disease is the one a patient loses oneself, and devastates one's whole family. The cause of senile dementia is known to be the degeneration of brain nerves influenced by abnormal protein. The degeneration of brain nerve cells and the pollution of synapse are influenced by the toxins produced in stomach and intestines. This is the reason why there are more Alzheimer's disease among chronic constipation patients and gastrointestinal tract disorder patients.

Brain nerve cell degeneration can be prevented through the treatment of phlegm mass disorder. By removing the wastes in the area of synapse, we may accomplish the normal response of brain nerve cells.

Treating diabetes becomes easy

Diabetes is dangerous because of complications. More cases are reported when insulin therapy and medication therapy fail to lower blood sugar and preventing complication is not done properly. It is because diet habit is not improved and therefore phlegm mass disorder takes place. As is proven in the clinical case, if wastes in the tissue cell membrane removed, blood glucose can easily flow into the tissue cell membrane and its use of glucose increase and naturally blood sugar drops. This way is to increase blood glucose management capacity just by improving body condition. Then one can stop or reducing the medication and will eventually reach the fundamental treatment.

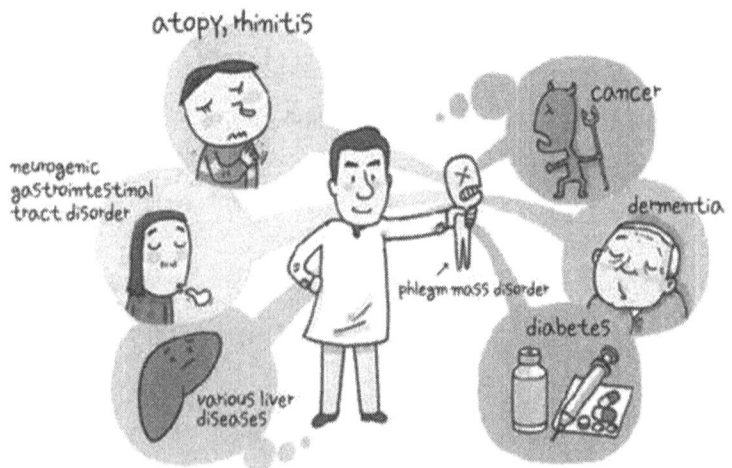

Stopping the evil cycle of children's cold, rhinitis, sinusitis, and atopy

Children's cold, rhinitis, sinusitis, and atopy do not leave them and continue to afflict them. The evil cycle of the disease will burden the health of children who will take us to the future. Medical insurance fund may collapse with this pace, we wonder. The problem is that many of these diseases originate from phlegm mass toxins. Phlegm mass toxins, when accumulated in nasal mucosa or in throat lymphatic system, bacteria will grow naturally in the mucosa. It will degenerate the immune response and inflammation take place often. When phlegm mass toxins overflows and exposes to the skin, with the accumulation of the toxin there, it creates degeneration of the skin and blood circulation disorder and forms atopy.

Phlegm mass issue may inherit from parents, but children nowadays, not like in the past, take toxin infested instant or fast foods. That's why children have lots of phlegm mass toxins these days. Knowing that these are eventually toxin originated, by removing phlegm mass toxins, purifying lymphatic function of upper respiratory tract, and removing of the accumulated toxins in the skin, we may accomplish fundamental treatment as well as greatly achieve prevention of the disease.

Way of treating neurogenic, hypersensitive gastro-intestinal disorder is opening

Since the cause of neurogenic indigestion and hypersensitive colon disorder is proved to be phlegm mass disorder, the fundamental treatment of them is possible. Not being detected over endoscopy, various gastrointestinal disorders were classified as neurogenic or hypersensitive, but not anymore. We do not need to use the words, 'neurogenic' or 'hypersensitive,' and its treatment will be easy, we expect.

Treatment of intractable autoimmune disease is possible

Intractable diseases such as Behcet's disease, lupus disease, are rheumatoid arthritis becomes curable through the phlegm mass disorder treatment.

Autoimmune diseases is not what outside germs invade in and cause disease, but antigen being made inside and to remove this, immune response created and making friendly fight, like the civil war between the north and the south going on. Modern medicine finds it difficult to understand why this kind of abnormal immune war should take place. Oriental medicine explains that the antigen substance that causes autoimmune response has something to do with the environment of stomach, intestines, and liver. If the environment is dirty, germs and viruses will appear by themselves. This works as antigen and lead to work as immune response. In other words, the phlegm mass toxins cause pollution of the environment of stomach and intestines. If the phlegm mass toxin is treated, the antigen is not produced and therefore it becomes fundamentally changed.

For helpless cirrhosis and liver cancer, phlegm mass disorder treatment is the solution

Phlegm mass toxin flows into liver through portal vein and pollute liver environment and may worsen the liver damage. Therefore transfer from hepatitis to cirrhosis depends completely on gastrointestinal tract status. Oriental medicine explains that gastrointestinal tract status can transfer to liver as it is, and liver and cirrhosis are even called 'the disease of the stomach.' Recently, more virus-related hepatitis patient cases transfer to cirrhosis. It is because the degeneration of middle zone toxin causes the environment pollution in those organs. Improving middle zone environment by removing phlegm mass toxins, letting clean blood flow into the liver, not the polluted one, we can then minimize the malign kinds of liver diseases.

For uterine diseases, bladder and prostate diseases, healing and prevention is possible with medication without having to undergo surgery

Various uterine diseases such as leukorrhea, intrauterine infection, and uterine myoma also take place when phlegm mass toxins flow in and set in the uterine walls. It causes bacteria increase and growth of uterine lining. Especially the women's bladder diseases such as frequent cystitis, frequent urination, and urinary incontinence also look connected to phlegm mass disorder. If Cajal cells that exist in smooth muscles and control the movements of bladder damaged by phlegm mass toxins, the tissues of the bladder hardened and mobility decreased. It will then cause to have frequent need to urinate, feeling incomplete, and have cystitis easily.

In clinical practices, when phlegm mass disorder treatment was administered to smooth muscle related diseases such as uterine myoma and frequent urination, and cystitis, and to the patients of enlarged prostate, many positive results have been reported. This proves that phlegm mass toxins cause uterine myoma, bladder disease, and prostate disease. And the toxins come from degenerated gastrointestinal tract.

Musculoskeletal disorder prevention is possible

Intramuscular pain happens because of phlegm mass disorder. Shoulders, nape of the neck, and back become hardened and pain appears because, in most cases, phlegm mass get accumulated in the muscles and cause the pain. Other musculoskeletal disorders in waist and legs are also influenced by phlegm mass and get hardened. Muscle operates because of the blood supplied from stomach, intestines, and liver. If the muscle receives phlegm mass toxins, it becomes hardened and swells up, and may cause motor disturbance and pain to appear often. In clinical cases, the removing of phlegm mass from musculoskeletal disorder can result in relaxing of muscles and reducing pains. This may show the relationship between muscle disorder and phlegm mass disorder.

TIP: Splanchnic nerve's codification of food

The nerve codifies the master's favorite food and remembers it. When the food comes in, it allows free pass. If the food is of good quality, fine, if not, whole body may become worse. If kids are used to instant or fast food, they will not eat good food such as kimchi or bean paste stew, and find only codified bad foods. That's why when Koreans visit USA they crave for eating kimchi.

Part 07

Silencing the Revolt of Food Container

1
Time to examine our unusual eating habits!

It is time to put Koreans' unusual eating habits on the table and talk about them. It is not only about indigestion issue, but also about how the eating habits and eating cultures of us raise chronic and serious problems in our gastrointestinal tract and the whole body. The combination of unhealthy culture and our ignorance on the medical & science concerns on the issues have left the nation to countless number of diseases. With the rapid development of petroleum industry especially after the 20th century, serious environmental pollution spread and our table is no longer safe. Because of the pollution of water and soil, the foods we used to regard them good hurt us with their toxins instead. Despite the enormous advancement of the modern medicines, cancer rate and death rate are ever increasing. Those chronic, intractable, and adult diseases such as diabetes, cirrhosis, high blood pressure, stroke, various skin diseases, and thyroid disease rapidly and comfortably set in our body. However, medical cause analysis has not completed yet for all these dilemmas, and those are not irrelevant to pollution of the dining table, we feel.

New medical insights recently suggest that all these diseases may have originated from wrong health care and toxin issues. With the discovery of phlegm mass disorder, new medical theories about chronic, intractable, malign diseases, along with eating issues will likely to appeal to us. As Hippocrates said, the father of western medicine, 'a disease food cannot cure, neither will doctors,' food will be in the center of prevention and treatment of all disease.

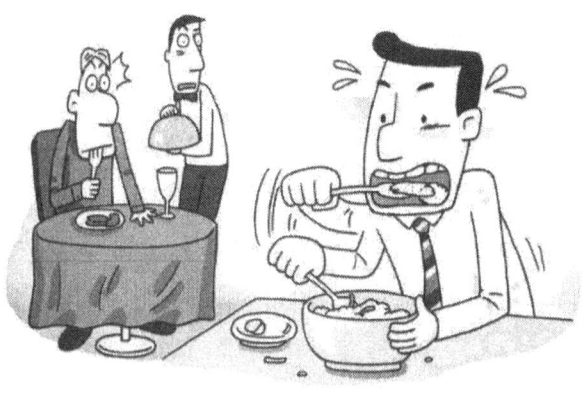

It is time to acknowledge that eating is important, but what and how to eat is more important. We have to completely change the way we recklessly treat the gastrointestinal tract as food container. Even when eating a spoonful of rice, we have to consider the stomach who would receive it 10 seconds later. 'Food container will handle it, of course!' With this kind of indifferent attitude of ours, stomach suffers from inexpressible hardship. Even a fly has its anger. Even a worm will turn. Likewise, our food container will not bear with us all the way. We don't know what the angry food container will do to us.

2

Foods and eating habits that easily cause phlegm mass disorder

Physical stimulus

Overeating, sporadic overeating, fast eating, eating cold food, vomit, and reflux inflict direct and physical damage not only the mucous membrane of gastrointestinal tract but also the muscle and nervous system, create lots of undigested substances, and make the environment dirty inside. Digestive enzymes mostly work on the surface of the food. When chunk of food lowered to the stomach, not all of them resolved, and some chyme remain in the stomach and produce toxins. These unresolved chyme and toxins eventually permeate the gastrointestinal tract outer wall, and create phlegm mass there.

Chemical stimulus

Salty or sweet food, antibiotic medicine or painkiller, strong acid or alkaline food, alcohol, flour, meat, and polluted food damage outer walls of gastrointestinal tract mucous membrane and create chemical change.

Biological stimulus

Foods influence the distribution of normally residing germs in the gastrointestinal tract. When the harmful and good bacteria become unbalanced, diverse diseases appear. Lactic acid bacteria, Helicobacter, and E.coli are among the well-known bacteria.

TIP: A phenomenon: drinking water in other places when traveling causes diarrhea

The mechanism of changing water causes diarrhea when traveling is not completely explained yet. It is roughly understood that a particular signal transmitter is activated in the intestine epithelial cell, and intestine permeability increased before causing the diarrhea. In oriental medicine, the absorption of nutrition and moisture in small and large intestines can perform properly only when liver metabolism functions well. However, when liver's function freezes because of stress, disorder happens in metabolism and moisture absorption is not done, rather moisture gets out and diarrhea happens. In oriental medicine, it is called 'disharmony between the liver and the spleen.'

3

Health care guide that silences all diseases

Avoid overeating, sporadic overeating, and fast eating

'The most foolish thing in the world is to sacrifice health to gain a certain profit.' E. Spencer, the English poet, remarked. As life expectancy prolongs, wellbeing food has gained more attention. Along with what to eat, how to eat can never be overemphasized. According to the 'national health and nutrition in depth analysis report' done by Korea Institute for Health and Social Affairs, Koreans' life expectancy was 78.6 year old on the basis of 2005, but the healthy life expectancy that life without diseases/disorders was 68.6 year old (men 67.4, women 69.6). The 10 years of finishing year is accompanied by various kinds of unfortunate diseases. How can we, then, prolong healthy life expectancy?

In the midst of busy life, we are used to the bad habit of fast eating, overeating, and sporadic overeating. When eating fast, we will have undigested food wastes and those will destroy the mucous membrane, in the middle zone, the protector of our health. When we eat much, in order to digest, oxygen demand gets increased, more active oxygen produced and therefore cells and DNA get damaged. We don't have this concept in mind and live in wrong dining cultures as if eating fast is a virtue.

We now have to develop the wise dining culture to protect the gastrointestinal tract mucous membrane healthy and not to have toxins such as active oxygen or wastes inside of us.

333 eating habit campaign

For healthy life, we will need to strive to chew our food well. We may not be able to spend 1 or 2 hours for having meal as some people of developed countries do. In order to raise the health index, we hope to spread the 333 eating habit campaign.

It is to have 3 meals a day regularly, to chew 30 times a mouth to mix with saliva, and to spend 30 minutes a meal. We will have to spread this new dining table culture from home to work. Treating slow eaters as fools or pressing others to eat faster should be stopped. Instead, we will have to make the dining a time to talk and to enjoy eating slowly. In case it is really urgent occasion and need to eat fast, we may want to put more portion in the mouth and mix with saliva and chew it fast. If we practice 333 eating habit campaign thoroughly, we may noticeably feel that our health becomes better.

Cook your rice mushy and eat small

Make your rice watery and eat small portion as much as possible. Those with serious phlegm mass disorder case, it is especially better to have the rice watery. Avoid multi-grain rice such as unpolished rice, bean, or red bean for some time. Avoid also the rice cooked in pressure cooker, rice cake, and even small bit of flour dishes. It is easy to digest porridge, mashed potatoes, and soft boiled eggs. Hard-boiled rice, spicy cold chewy noodles, black-bean-sauce noodles, fried foods are not easy to digest. It should be the norm for the phlegm mass disorder patients to have balanced nutrition and of easy to digest. It is not easy to suggest ideal amount of food for all the people because of individual differences. But it is always good to take only 70% of one's full portion. Even for the sake of eating small portion, it is good to get used to chew for a long time. Eating food fast, we may not feel the taste of the food enough and just swallow. Since we don't feel the taste enough, we try to satisfy the desire by eating much. Besides, it takes some time for stomach to feel the sense of satisfaction. If eating fast, therefore, we may have overeaten already before brain feels the satisfaction.

Steam it or boil it

Our stomach likes to have soft cooked foods such as boiled or steamed ones. Even for people without phlegm mass disorder, this kind of food is good for health. When eating meat, if it is boiled, the fat better be removed, and then we eat low fat and high protein. No matter how good material we use, once fried in oil, much nutrition get damaged and cause the obesity. Blue-backed fish is the same. The fish fat and oil can be easily oxidized and can inflict harm to body. How to cook is very important.

Avoid late-night meal and do not go to bed right after the meal

Eating just before going to bed is to make food wastes in the stomach. Habitual eating late-night meal is a common cause of visceral fat. These people usually have thick phlegm mass layer inside. With the serious phlegm mass, reflux easily happens and develops to reflux esophagitis. Continuous accumulation of phlegm mass toxins will directly result in stomach cancer, colon cancer, myoma, skin diseases, and obesity. Avoid late-night meal no matter what! Neither do going to bed immediately after the meal. It takes roughly 4 hours to digest food. Therefore we have to finish taking food 4 or 5 hours before going to bed. It is good to refrain from going to bed in 2 hours after the meal.

* *Foods easily causing stomach upset*

Boiled sweet potato, rice cake, apple, shrimp, cuttle fish, sushi, corn, ramen, black-bean-sauce noodles, flour dish such as bread, stir-fried-glass noodles, raw fish, fast food, instant food, and red bean dish etc.

* *Good food*

Kimchi, soybean stew, seasoned vegetables, green vegetables, mung beans, seaweeds, fish, persimon leaf tea, and black bean, etc.

Sugar is especially bad!

Sugar is bad, because it relaxes gastrointestinal mucous membrane and lowers the stomach acid. It therefore raises the permeability of wastes to middle zone, causes visceral fat, weakens the immune capacity of gastrointestinal tract, and prompts to increase the bad bacteria. In addition to this, it accumulates fat in the body, gain weight, and sharply raise the concentration of neutral fat of the blood.

Keep away from carbonated drinks

The carbonated drinks may give us temporary relief when eating fat foods, but it does not do any good to stomach. The carbonated drink has lots of fruit sugar in it and it is not absorbed in stomach or in small intestine. Rather, it flows down to large intestine. In the process, it produces gas and make it feeling bloating. To this gas, the gas from carbonated drink added and it impedes the intestinal contraction and pollutes the intestinal environment, and makes it the breeding ground of various diseases.

Drink alcohol moderately

Alcohol can penetrate the mucous membrane of the gastrointestinal tract better than any kind of food does. Drinking moderate amount of alcohol can help blood circulation and promote activating energy. But too much consumption of it damages the mucous membrane and therefore destroys the middle zone. It also worsens the liver function that it does not detoxicate various kinds of poisons and cause the toxins spread all over the body.

Eat foods with sulfur dioxide

Active oxygen is known to break up gastrointestinal tract mucous membrane and to cause many different kinds of whole body diseases. Eat vegetables and fruits that contain lots of sulfur dioxide to prevent from damaging middle zone. If it is not enough with vegetables and fruits, take sulfur dioxide vitamins and minerals in addition.

Stop smoking

No more explanation is needed for this issue. To put one more reason, cigarette produces active oxygen and accelerates aging process, and cause fatal diseases such as cancers and arteriosclerosis. Just by not smoking, we may extend life expectancy by 10 years.

Manage stress immediately

People of good stress manager may live average 16 years more than those who are not, according to a research. As mentioned earlier, stress produces strong poisonous stress hormones and increases aggressive substances such as stomach acid, mastocyte, and histamine. They not only damage gastrointestinal tract mucous membrane but also damage blood vessel, good body fluids, and DNA inside cells, the basic structure of whole body. Stress can be also the basis of all diseases. It is therefore important to calm down angered emotion by ways of hobby, travel, yoga, abdominal breathing, religious life, and meditation. When stressed out, not losing calmness, but maintaining pleasant and smiling response to stresses is important.

Regulated life is the basics of life

We have biological clock in our body. To follow the order of this biological clock is the key to live long. The people of longevity have something in common; they lived regulated life.

Do light exercise steadily

Steady physical activities are necessary. Phlegm mass disorders are among the people of little physical activities. Low intensity exercise such as jogging, stretching, walking, swimming, climbing upstairs, and mountain climbing, is better than high intensity ones. If the exercise becomes too much of burden, it does not do any good but harms us. If the phlegm mass symptom is advanced, it is better not to do the exercise intensely. Doing exercise is good if it is done 2 hours after mealtime.

TIP: Diarrhea, the unwanted guest who comes anytime!

Diarrhea is when one often defecates and the waste becomes

watery, sometimes even like water. There are many different reasons for diarrhea and the mechanisms of it are as follows.

1) When there are lots of high molecular or not absorbed substances in the large intestine, by the osmotic pressure effect, moistures from intestines tract come out to inside the intestine and cause the diarrhea. Osmotic pressure diarrhea is caused by overeating or sporadic overeating.
2) When inflammation or ulcer is formed in the mucous membrane of large intestine, its moisture absorption capacity gets damaged and diarrhea suddenly takes place. If mucous membrane becomes severely damaged and mucus or blood oozes out, mucous stool or blood accompanies. Inflammation or ulcer happens when there is spicy food or untreated toxins.
3) Large intestine's absorption capacity functions well when it is dry and warm inside, oriental medicine says. The absorption capacity entirely depends on Yang (plus) energy. If large intestine is cold, it cannot absorb the moisture because the nature of water is Yin (minus) energy, then diarrhea happens. Diarrhea when eating raw and cold food, diarrhea in the early morning, and diarrhea with pain in the lower abdomen when stressed out all belong to this category. This kind of diarrhea is called of deficiency of the *Yang* of the spleen and the kidney.

If large intestine is wet, it does not absorb moisture. Instead, it expels moisture out of mucous membrane and then stool becomes hard. If it is wet, pathological bacteria increase easily and diarrhea happens. The reason large intestinal environment becomes wet like swamp is because of untreated chyme, because of overeating and excess taking of meats, flow into large intestine and delay there or taking too much alcohol and unabsorbed moisture get mixed with food wastes and create wet environment. Intestines by nature do not like moisture. That's why diarrhea happens more often when eating food with lots of water or in the rainy season.

4) Excess exasperation of intestinal movement can also cause diarrhea. Excess exasperation of vermicular movements is caused by severe stress, overeating, sporadic overeating, and surgical removal of gastrointestinal tract. Diarrhea caused by overeating is a natural nervous physiological reaction to protect against the big amount of food wastes damaging our body. Once removing the food, we will not have much problem. When diarrhea is caused by severe stress, oriental medicine explains that heat natured energy of liver causes it. Severe stresses such as anger or shock form strong heat natured energy and it is called transverse flow of the liver energy (Qi). If the energy should attack intestine, the intestinal muscle causes spasm and diarrhea takes place. When feeling intestine twisted inside and have diarrhea because of the stress, it is caused by the energy of the liver.

Appendix

I treated my gastrointestinal tract this way

'Once swallowing something, my pit of the stomach became dead blocked, my brain got bloated, and I could not do anything.'

Name: Yon Ju Na

Major symptoms: amnesia, declining of eyesight, phlegm, asthenia, insomnia, chronic migraine, suffocating, feeling something in the throat, frequent stomach upset, heartburn, constipation, and neurogenic gastritis.

I suffered from indigestion, constipation, heartburn, and migraine for 20 years and literally lived on digestive medicine and constipation medicine. When receiving endoscopy once a year, I was diagnosed as having 'neurogenic gastritis' and was given gastritis medication and mostly tranquilizer and was asked about my relationship with my husband and that with his family. I faithfully took the gastritis medication but did not improve much. If I should eat something, my pit of the stomach became dead blocked, my brain got bloated, and I could not do anything. Out of desperation, I had my son press on the spot, pit of the stomach, with his heel for 20 to 30 minutes massage on my shoulders, and poke the nape of my neck with a ball pen point. If it was not enough, I ran for massage shop to relieve my abdomen and to massage the whole body. I had MRI scan because of the chronic migraine, but nothing was proven wrong.

In the recent years, along with the menopause the following symptoms made the quality of my life miserable; amnesia, declining of eyesight, phlegm that I spit continually, asthenia, insomnia, chronic migraine, suffocating, feeling something in the throat, and frequent stomach upset. I felt sad and depressed, the whole body and mind. I lacked energy and very much worried. At that time, I knew that an aunt of my husband's side was visiting Weedahm Oriental Hospital, and the phlegm mass disorder I read was addressing my disease. I immediately made an appointment and started taking medication for 10 days. After taking it for 3 days, to my surprise, I started feeling comfortable inside. Believing that I would be better if I had intensified the treatment, I got hospitalized. Being admitted to the hospital, I fasted for 5 days. 2 days after the beginning of the fasting, the severe back pain of mine began to relieve, heartburn reduced, headache disappeared, whole body became as light as feather, suffocating feeling stopped that I took a deep and short breath alternatively to appreciate the positive change of my body.

After finishing the fasting, I started taking thin rice porridge and carefully examine my body; my back pain became weaker and weaker, heartburn completely disappeared, I did not need any constipation medicine anymore to go to the restroom, phlegm stopped, the feeling of something stuck in my throat disappeared, ugly looking benign tumor in the nape of my neck diminished much. All these were amazing change to me.

During those phlegm mass removing therapies, I was doubtful about food stagnancy removal therapy and aroma therapy. 'Do I have to receive these therapies?' I wondered and questioned a lot to the nurses of the therapies and sought the responses from other patients. But I now feel very much grateful to Dr. Choi for the development of the therapy. And besides, combination of physical therapy and herb medicine solved the problem of phlegm mass disorder of mine. Since my aunt began to get well and I too experienced this much fast treatment, I would like to share my experience of treatment with anyone who have suffered from the phlegm mass disorder and invite them to Weedahm Oriental Hospital.

'To those who have tried various treatments but still suffer from pains, I would say that phlegm mass disorder treatment is the miraculous one!'

Name: Min Jin Kim

Major symptoms: headache, coldness of body, insomnia, gastrospasm, reflux esophagitis, gastrorrhagia, dry eyeness, rhinitis, constipation, diarrhea, shoulders and back pain, indigestion, heartburn, chronic fatigue, chest pain, feeling something stuck in the throat
Surgical operation received: large intestine, small intestine, gallbladder, appendectomy

I often had headache, whole body being cold, suffered insomnia, gastrospasm, reflux esophagitis, gastrorrhagia, eye dryness, rhinitis, constipation, having severe pain on shoulders and right side back feeling uncomfortable when lying down on bed, and whatever I ate, it caused upset stomach easily. I underwent all available tests and treatments in internal medicine. No medication and injection worked. Ordinary oriental medicine clinics did not help me either. I also visited and received different kinds of treatments from pain clinics, ENT clinics, and ophthalmic clinic. Each time I visited those clinics, those medications I was given made inside of me even more painful.

Not eating properly, having not enough sleep, my body went wrong in all directions, and I had some part of my large intestine, small intestine, gallbladder, and appendix removed. Treatments became even more difficult. Liver and heart became worse, not to speak of stomach. I felt always tired and chest was stiff. I sometimes felt difficult to breath. I did not know what treatments I should take further from there.

After I visited Weedahm Oriental Hospital, my life has become different; cold body of mine much warmer, Headache disappeared, rhinitis eased, feeling something stuck in my throat gone, sense of heartburn stopped, and the hardened stomach softened. I feel something has gotten away from there. I started eating meal and make some sleep more and more. I have become more comfortable at every passing day and I feel happy.

I remember the time when I first received the aroma therapy and food stagnancy removal therapy. There was a lot of water stirring sound. I felt something is passing through the intestines. I farted a lot and made sleep long time for the first time. I felt very light later. While hospitalized, I experienced different symptoms repeated appearing and my body becoming changed. The phlegm mass on stomach part eventually resolved and I am now surprisingly treated.

To those who have tried various treatments but still suffer from pains, I would say that phlegm mass disorder treatment is the miraculous one! I thought I would have no hospital to treat my diseases, but I came across the fortune. Dr. Seo Hyung Choi, the director of Weedahm Oriental Hospital, discovered the new disease, phlegm mass disorder, and treats patients with various medications and equipment. I am now given new opportunity of living. Those who now suffer from this disease, start having this treatment with hope! Each day will be filled with happiness. Cheer up, please! Go for it!

'I felt that I could be healed. With the hope, the cloud of depression scattered.'

Name: Yon Ju Do

Major symptoms: calcific tendinitis of shoulders, neck/waist disc, phlegm mass disorder, fibromyositis, and anaplastic arthritis

When eating something, I felt indigestion to the point of feeling something stuck in the throat, feeling pain on back, shoulders, and the head, having difficulties in breathing, chronic fatigue, and lethargy. I underwent endoscopy in two different clinics with no results. With medication, I still felt uneasiness in my stomach. I also had acupuncture treatment and phlegm mass disorder treatment in an oriental clinic in Daegu, a city in Korea, with no result except for less frequent burp. Indigestion continued. Just taking a spoonful of western medicine made my stomach bloating and painful that I could not take the medication anymore. Taking vitamin C or other nutritional supplements caused indigestion that I could not continue.

At one point, I came across the Weedahm Oriental Hospital and visited once. I thought 'this is it!' When I had 2 weeks of hospital treatment, I saw the hope there. I felt that I could be healed. With the hope, the cloud of depression scattered. I decided to put my trust in Dr. Choi and followed the treatment. With such a positive attitude, I felt the improvements. I used to feel that something is clogged from my back to shoulder and to neck. Breathing was hard back then. It became easier and the pain in the back and the shoulders has become much relieved. The suffocating feeling in the pit of the stomach and the pounding of heartbeat are much relieved. Headache is almost gone. The backs of thighs' tingling feeling and the coldness of heel are much improved.

Medical staff of Weedahm Oriental Hospital has been lots of comfort to me when hospitalized because of the pains. It worked positively in treating the diseases. I expressed my gratitude to each and every one of the staff including acupuncture therapists, aroma therapists, food stagnancy removal therapist, moxibustion therapist, and all the nurses. Being sensitive to cold, Korean style sauna that is made of yellow soil was my favorite place. It meant more than just treatment.

I was depressed as I went about western/oriental hospitals, because I became worse at every passing date. Extreme fatigue and lethargy of mine deprived me of the joy of life. After I began receiving the hospital treatment, I became confident of the complete recovery. The gradual improvement of the shoulders and the backs, restoration of digesting ability, escaping from the headaches and from lethargy, all these gave me sense of happiness.

When I eat food, I chew more than 40 times each mouthful. It made me digest food better and feel the preciousness of the food. With small amount of food, I could feel satisfied. I remember I wasted lots of food. For those who are suffering from phlegm mass disorder, there is hope of treatment! Do not hesitate to start the treatment, and start it now!

'I now have confidence of living healthier than anybody else.'
Name: Kyung Wha Yoon

Major symptoms: gastritis, chronic stomach ulcer, indigestion, stomachache, bloating, depression, rhinitis, insomnia, cystitis, and hypernoia

From gastritis to stomach ulcer, I always had internal medicine treatment. I underwent endoscopy and received helicobacter treatment. I was prescribed with stomach ulcer treatment for 2 months at a time, but feeling pain in the stomach, I did not have improvement no matter how hard I took the medications. Smelling food was difficult that I became very nervous about whether I would contract a big disease. Lower abdomen was always bloating. Having indigestion problem, the abdomen did not retrieve no matter how hard I diet. I suffered severe stomachache because of the depression 2 years ago. For that, I received treatment in the neuropsychiatric clinic for 6 months. But I did not feel any improvements at that time. I later knew Weedahm Oriental Hospital and got examined there. Though I heard about the 'phlegm mass disorder' for the first time, I decided to trust Dr. Choi and got hospitalized. As soon as I got accepted, liver purification treatment started, I felt my head became sparkling fresh clean. It was like I became of my early 30s. Undergoing food stagnancy removing therapy, I felt all my intestinal organs began to move and make sounds. It was surprising. I felt that the aching parts of my body became better at every passing date. Breathing became much easier. Smelling food was much better. The body and the head became light, the dimming eyesight brighter, and the depressed mindset cleared, Insomnia better and rhinitis disappeared. When feeling tired, I used to suffer from cystitis, but it is OK now. While hospitalized, I was always busy with taking medications and receiving different kinds of treatments, I am now leaving this hospital with healthy body. I now have confidence to live healthier than anybody else. Thank you! Lastly, for those who suffer from chronic indigestion, always carrying digestive medicine, who think that they just have to carry the unknown disease, suffering the pain but no one around understand them, and undergoing depression because of the symptoms, come to Weedahm Oriental Hospital and receive the treatment!

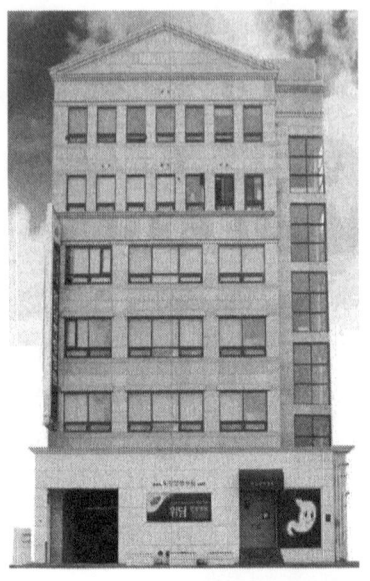

Weedahm Oriental Hospital at Seoul

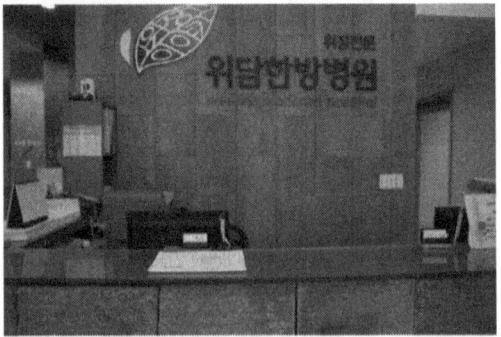

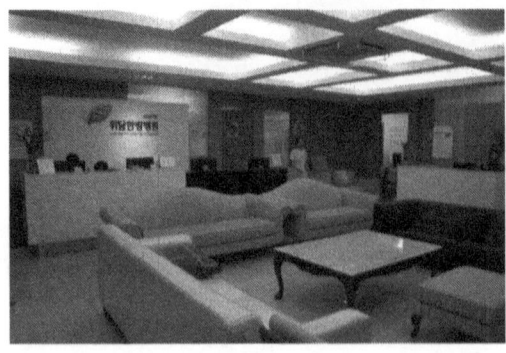

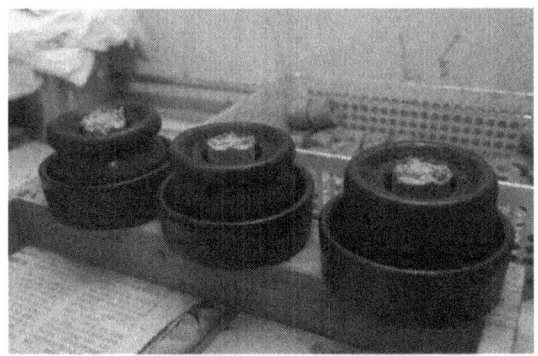

Moxibustion

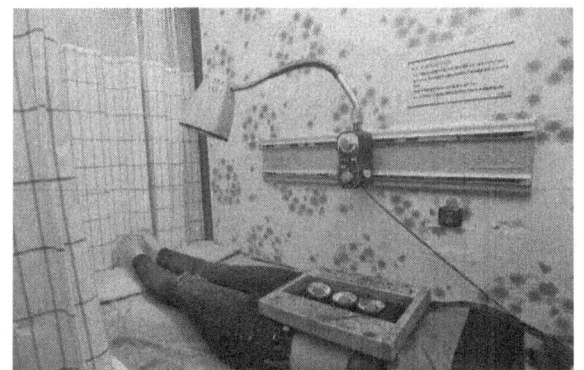

Moxibustion Therapy

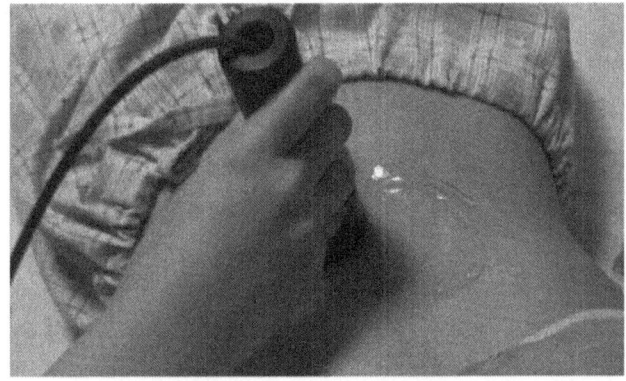

Ultrasonic Therapy

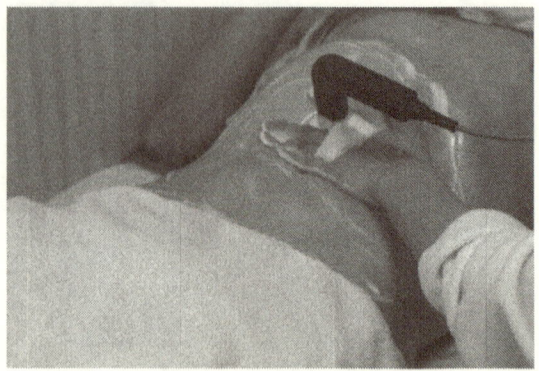

Aroma Therapy

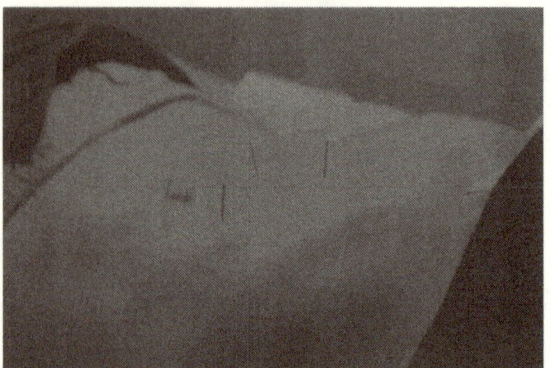

Herbal Acupuncture Therapy

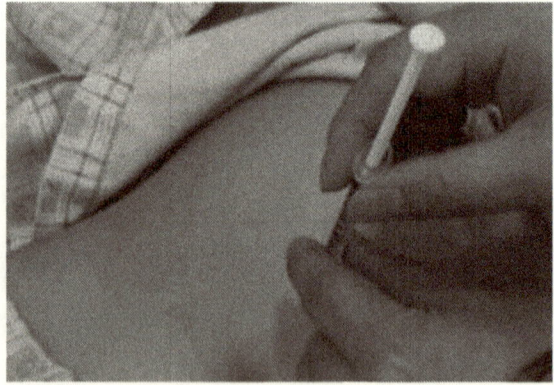

Herbal Acupuncture Therapy

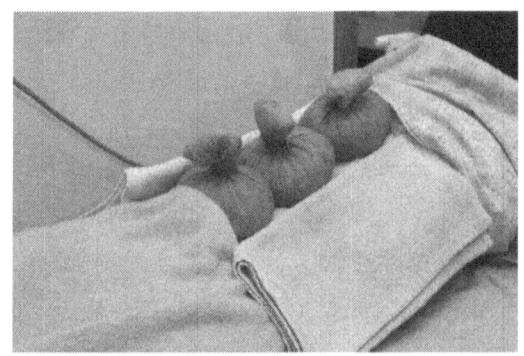

Treatment with Heat of Steamed Herbs

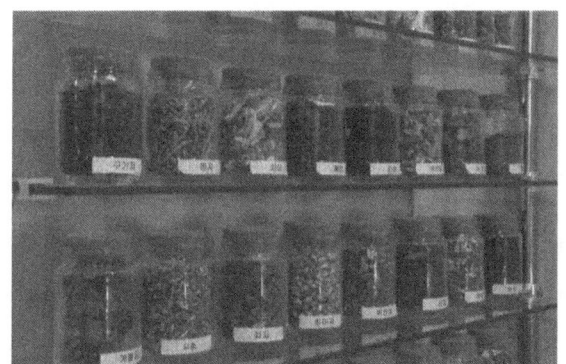

Medicinal Herbs

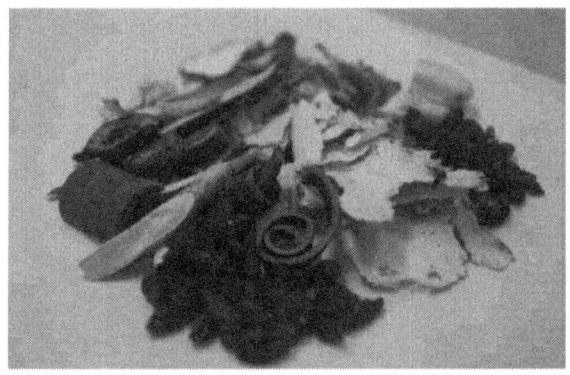

Medicinal Herbs

Translator's Note

For years, my wife suffered from painful digestive issues of unknown cause with various accompanying symptoms that gradually emaciated her until she was a fraction of her former weight. Since she met Dr. Choi at Weedahm Oriental Hospital, however, she has begun to recover from such horrible gastrointestinal tract disorders. Out of the sheer gratitude that we have felt for helping her out of her plight, I picked up the book 'Revolt of The Stomach' that was written by him and began to translate it into English for the benefit of an English speaking audience, who are unfamiliar with his work.

In order to translate the book, I had to read the text from cover to cover. By the time I had finished it, the entire content of the book had been boiled down to a simple truth before me that our health heavily depends on what we eat and how we eat it. Once I had truly understood this point and began to live by it, reaping its benefits, I feel as though I no longer need to seek the help of medicine, as the key to a healthy life for most of us is simply good healthy living.

Dr. Kong, Choon Taeck

About the Translator

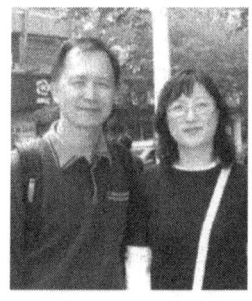 Dr. Kong, Choon Taeck has been teaching English composition in universities in China and in Kazakhstan since 2002. He is married to Kyung-Hee, and is a proud father of a daughter through whom he has further been blessed with four grandsons. Kong received BA degree from Seoul Theological University in 1980, Doctor of Ministry from Claremont University in 2002, and Honorary Doctorate (Doctor of Divinity) from Asbury Theological Seminary in 2002. He served in cross cultural projects since 1992, founded Kazakhstan Evangelical Christian Seminary in 1993 and served as President until 2005, taught in Xinjiang University of Finance and Economics as a Professor of English from December 2002 till July 2009, served as a visiting scholar at Drew University from September 1, 2006 to June 1, 2007, taught English composition at the University of Electronic Science of Technology of China from March 2011 until Spring 2016, and taught MBA and Professional English at Kazakh British Technical University (KBTU) in Fall 2016 semester.

Email: kongyoung53@yahoo.com

About the Author

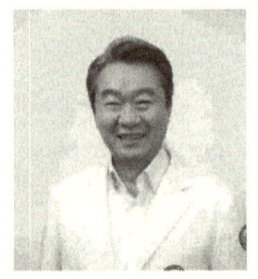 Dr. Seo Hyung Choi is the director and chairman of the board of trustee of Weedahm Oriental Hospital, chairman of Korea Global Medical Industry Research Society, adjunct professor of Kyunghee Oriental & Western Medicine Graduate School; chairman of the Society of Phlegm Mass Syndrome, chairman of New Way New Mission, Corp., chairman of board of trustees of Natural Healing Tourism Forum. He graduated from undergraduate and graduate school of Kyunghee Oriental Medicine University and acquired a master and a doctorate degree (majored in Liver and Internal Medicine), completed top management course (1st class) of Health Graduate School of Seoul National University. He served as a clinical professor at Kyunghee Oriental Medicine University affiliated Hospital (Oriental & Western Medicine Research Center), head professor of Oriental Medicine College of Daejeon University, adjunct professor of Oriental Medicine College of Dongguk University, adjunct Professor of Yonsei University at Wonju Campus, and the first chairman of Consolidated Cancer Research Center. He founded the first combined Western & Oriental Medicine Hospital in South Korea in 1992 and was awarded the first Medical doctor with New Intelligence of Republic of Korea Award.

Website: weedahm.com | Email: hana9212@korea.com

www.ingramcontent.com/pod-product-compliance
Lightning Source LLC
Chambersburg PA
CBHW031052180526
45163CB00002BA/803